'Michael Crossland is truly one is, at times, heart wrenching, but the overarching message of refusing to let adversity define you struck a chord with our audience that I don't believe we have hit before, or will manage to again. Never have I seen 500 people leap to their feet so quickly in a unified standing ovation. As a professional speaker, Michael's attention to detail, ability to speak to brief and skill with an audience's focus, was second to none. From a booking point of view, he was friendly, approachable and entirely focused on what we were trying to achieve at our event. I cannot recommend him enough.'

Stephanie Wells — Marketing Communications Manager, Franchise Council of Australia

'Words escape me to truly express my thanks for the amazing journey you took us all on today as the keynote speaker at the HR Teams event in Sydney and the roller-coaster ride of emotions you evoked in us all. I feel incredibly humbled and honoured to have met you and want you to know how much you touched everyone in the room today (myself included) with your warmth, passion, incredible spirit and courage in the face of such adversity.

The room was charged full of raw energy and emotion when you finished, and many members commented to me afterwards how incredibly inspirational you were and how powerful your messages, learnings and insights were. My congratulations.

I feel very privileged to have met you and wish you well on your continued inspirational journey.'

Amanda McKernan — Director, International HR Director Forum, CEO Forum Group

'Thank you for sharing your inspiring, yet very personal, story at our company Kick Start event earlier this year. From business to sport, you reminded us that in life anything we set our mind to we can accomplish successfully. You are a true inspiration to us all.'

**John McGrath — Chief Executive Officer,
McGrath Estate Agents**

'Thank you for joining us in Melbourne to share your incredible story with the team at Buxton. Your achievements in the face of adversity in both business and sport are truly remarkable. Hearing about your tenacity and persistence in the face of so many hurdles was inspirational and highly motivating for those of us who work in a competitive sales environment and have our wins and disappointments, albeit no comparison with yours. Perhaps your experience in sales and sales management helped, but we felt you connected particularly well with our people from the outset and the feedback since has been nothing short of exceptional. We are all better for the experience.'

**Gavan Fallon — Managing Director,
Buxton Real Estate Group Pty Ltd**

'The feedback from our leadership was fantastic, and after assessing the feedback sheets 100% of the delegates rated your session as Excellent! It was wonderful to have you share your story with our team again.'

**Olivia Walsh — Organisational Learning
& Development Manager, CBRE**

EVERYTHING WILL BE OK

EVERYTHING WILL BE OK

A STORY OF HOPE, LOVE AND PERSPECTIVE

MICHAEL CROSSLAND

WILEY

First published in 2020 by John Wiley & Sons Australia, Ltd
42 McDougall St, Milton Qld 4064
Office also in Melbourne

Typeset in Adobe Jenson Pro Regular 14/17.5pt by SPi Global, India

© John Wiley & Sons Australia, Ltd 2020

The moral rights of the author have been asserted

ISBN: 978-0-730-38501-1

A catalogue record for this book is available from the National Library of Australia

Cover design by Wiley
Author photos by Ben Adams

10 9 8 7 6 5 4 3 2 1

Disclaimer
The material in this publication is of the nature of general comment only, and does not represent professional advice. It is not intended to provide specific guidance for particular circumstances and it should not be relied on as the basis for any decision to take action or not take action on any matter which it covers. Readers should obtain professional advice where appropriate, before making any such decision. To the maximum extent permitted by law, the author and publisher disclaim all responsibility and liability to any person, arising directly or indirectly from any person taking or not taking action based on the information in this publication.

This book is dedicated to a lady who sacrificed so much in her life, a lady who walked away from her husband and three daughters for numerous years in order to instil love, optimism, courage and hope into a young life that was supposed to end far too soon.

I dedicate this emotional account of my life to my amazing mum, Kerri.

She inspired me to always work hard, to try my best and to never quit, regardless of what others may say!

Mum, you will forever be my mother, and you will forever remain the heart and soul of our family.

You have always taught us to shoot for the moon, and you constantly reminded us that even when we miss, we will still end up in the stars.

I am forever grateful for your belief that miracles do happen. I love you dearly, and even when the doctors said it was hopeless and to take me home to die, you never walked away. You have filled my soul with hope forever.

CONTENTS

Too often in life, people use their adversities as the reasons why they fail, instead of using their adversities as their motivation to succeed.

In Australian culture, heroes are often portrayed as sports people or millionaires. They might be a cricket player scoring a double century, a footballer scoring a hat-trick of several tries in one match, or an IT technician developing a new generation of smartphones, but the real heroes are those normal, everyday people who are faced with extreme challenges and adversity, but who never give up. They fight, they stand strong, and they come out on the other side with a smile on their face and a story to tell.

Michael Crossland is a prime example of a true hero. Michael faces extreme challenges every day of his life, but he stands tall and ensures that his courage and his positive outlook on life inspire other people across the world.

FOREWORD

Michael Crossland is one of the most inspiring and motivating people I have ever met. His resilience and optimism in the face of adversity is incredible and this book is a testament to his gratitude for life and determination to give back and serve others.

Through my 25 years in corporate life and being a CEO of a leading Australian public company, I have been fortunate to meet and have access to the best and brightest speakers around the world. Rarely have I met someone with the attitude like Michael to keep getting up when the world is telling them to stay down. I first met Michael at a dinner in Sydney full of corporate leaders and there was not a dry eye in the restaurant after hearing his moving and authentic life story of relentless optimism in the face of adversity.

Michael is now an international speaker and regularly presents to audiences over 5000 people. His ability to stir strong emotions, create positivity and motivation is life changing. I am grateful for the difference he has made to my team at Aventus. Despite his success as a speaker, author and an executive coach, he remains humble and I am blessed to call him not only a mentor but a lifelong friend.

In *Everything Will Be OK*, Michael shares the vulnerable and at times funny story of his journey, embedded with practical tools to shift your mindset. He demonstrates how to use adversity as a motivator to succeed versus an excuse to step back and be a victim. This book also provides an insight into a parent's unconditional love, hope and sacrifice for their child.

Michael is living proof that life is truly a gift and that anything is possible by dreaming big and taking daily action. His book is thought provoking and will leave you feeling in awe of his journey from surviving to thriving.

Darren Holland
CEO, Aventus Group

ABOUT THE AUTHOR

As one of Australia's most sought-after inspirational speakers, Michael has defied the odds of a life-threatening cancer to build his life of exceptional achievements.

He is a regular inspirational speaker for corporations, schools, professional sporting organisations and universities throughout the world. Michael has presented in front of over 600 000 people around the globe.

His journey has been shared on TV, including Fox Sports, ABC, Channel Seven and Nine Network, Full Potential TV, *The Get Inspired Project, Inspire Me Today* and countless radio shows throughout America, Fiji and Australia.

Along with the award-winning program about his life on *Australian Story*, Michael has also recently featured in a humanitarian documentary, *Hope for Haiti*, about the countless lives saved through the orphanage and school in Haiti with which he is involved.

Diagnosed with cancer before his first birthday and spending nearly a quarter of his life in hospital, doctors told him school and sport were not options. Infection and fatigue were too great a risk, and reaching his teenage years would be a miracle.

His only wish was to lead a normal life and be able to do all the things that other kids took for granted every day.

But he had a dream and an undying determination to achieve the impossible, irrespective of the size of the obstacles that lay ahead.

Now an accomplished businessman, National Ambassador for Camp Quality, Australian of the Year finalist, Australia Day Ambassador for eight consecutive years and International Hall of Fame inductee, Michael inspires people from all walks of life.

There is no doubt he has a heart for giving and a skill to engage people. He has gone from being one of the youngest State Development Managers for one of the largest companies in the world, to running five banks. He then left his finance career to follow his dreams in making a global impact, and he has certainly done that!

Michael's story 'Field of Dreams' was documented on *Australian Story* on ABC television. Through this documentary, his message touched the hearts of a nation; it's the story of how he overcame seemingly insurmountable obstacles to achieve success in both his personal and professional life.

INTRODUCTION

I am very blessed and privileged to live a wonderful life. I've had the chance to speak to the troops in Iraq who are fighting for our freedom. It hit home to me how much danger they face every day: I was supposed to actually fly to Iraq to speak, however, only weeks before my visit the base was under attack. So I was very grateful to be not only safe in Australia but also to have the technology to share my story from their base in Richmond, NSW. I have spent time with children in juvenile detention centres throughout the United States; a large proportion of these young kids, aged between 11 and 15, made just one bad decision, and, as a result, their freedoms and liberties were irrevocably withdrawn. It is almost impossible to comprehend the adversity that they have experienced for them to be branded criminals as mere children.

It begets the question: What type of environment were they raised in for them to consider their behaviour acceptable in any way, shape or form?

I have had the opportunity to spend time with the victims and families of the September 11 attacks of 2001. These people had their lives completely destroyed by an attack that was as abhorrent as it was unforeseen.

Yet, they still manage to get out of bed every single day of their lives, and they work hard to smile. Regardless of the pain, the suffering and the challenges that they continue to face, they still somehow manage to push through.

I was speaking to a gentleman about his experience as a victim of the September 11 attacks. He was working in one of the buildings on the 25th floor when it happened. He recalls being told to stay in his cubicle, to stay calm, and not move.

He went on to say: 'There was something telling me to get out, take the stairs and run.' He ran down 25 flights of stairs, and whilst in the stairwell, he heard a massive explosion and assumed that the building was about to crush him. Nevertheless, he kept running.

When he finally reached the ground floor, he ran outside, only to find what looked like a war zone. He looked over and saw that the explosion he heard earlier was the second tower, which had also been hit. He ran from the building and could hear loud, slapping noises.

He got far enough away, turned, and to his horror, he saw that the slapping noise was people hitting the pavement whilst trying to escape the burning building.

These stories are reminders to people that life is a gift; we need to embrace it and enjoy it while we can. Our lives can be turned upside down with just one phone call, one bad decision, one act of terror, and our lives may never be the same again.

I am a strong believer that it's not about the amount of years you live on this earth. Instead, what you fit into those years, how you help to make the world a better place, is what really matters.

There's a great proverb: 'I cried when I didn't get a new pair of shoes, until I saw a boy who had no feet.' I think it's very important that we develop a habit of stepping out of our own shoes to look at life through someone else's eyes.

This practice allows us to realise how lucky we are to have what we have. I think it's so important that we count our blessings instead of our problems.

Over the last few years, I've had numerous opportunities across the world to address large audiences as a speaker. There was one time that has truly changed my life forever.

I had married my high school sweetheart on 21 April and on 1 May I left the country for three months. I was going to travel around Australia for two months as a speaker, and then I was planning to go to the United States for a month. In those three months, I had scheduled just two days off, and in those two days I had planned to head back to Coffs Harbour to spend some time with my lovely wife.

About six weeks into the tour, I received a phone call from a lady in Adelaide. Her name was Michelle. She said to me:

'Michael, I heard you speak a couple of years ago. You really touched me. There's a young boy here in Adelaide. His name is Kai. He's been diagnosed with cancer.

We were wondering whether you could possibly donate your time, come out to Adelaide, and present and raise some money for the family because they're really struggling.'

I said: 'I'm pretty well booked out until September, but I'll come out when I return and I'll see how much money we can raise for this family.' It was all set. I was heading out there. Then, two weeks later, I received a phone call from a lady named Kylie who was also from Adelaide.

Kylie said to me, 'Michael, there's a young boy in Adelaide. His name is Kai. He's been diagnosed with cancer.'

I said, 'Yeah, I'm aware of him. I'm heading out there in September.'

She replied, 'Michael, Kai has just been transferred from the Oncology Ward to the Palliative Care Unit. This little five-year-old boy has less than two weeks to live, and his dying wish is to meet you.'

I am no superstar, no professional athlete, and nor am I a famous actor or hero. I stand here today as a man who has faced my fair share of adversity. Regardless, I continue to remember what Mum always told me: Irrespective of how many times you get knocked down, you just have to keep getting back up.

I called my wife and I told her about Kai. She said, 'Those two days you were going to spend with me: I want you to spend them with this little boy.'

I remember being on the plane flying to Adelaide from Sydney, and I said to myself: 'Don't emotionally connect with this little boy.' When I arrived in Adelaide, I got in a car and drove to the hospital. As I walked into the room, a little five-year-old boy ran across the floor and jumped into my arms. Instantly, I was emotionally connected with this little angel.

The little boy, his family and I all went out for a beautiful lunch and played catch. I gave him a few little gifts, and I let him steer the car back through the vineyards. He thanked me for a great day, and he told me that he would see me soon. I could not bring myself to say anything back, because I knew that I would never see that sweet little boy again.

That night, we raised thousands of dollars for the family, and the community's support was overwhelming. Sadly, little Kai was finished fighting, and three weeks later, while I was in the USA, I received a text message from his mum. The text read: 'My boy is cancer free and pain free.' My heart sank and tears flowed down my face unchecked, because of a heroic little boy who lost his battle with cancer.

Most of the money that had been raised to help Kai's family was used to bury beautiful Kai. The tears that continued to well in my eyes for many days after Kai passed away were not just of sadness; they were also tears of joy in the knowledge that I had experienced the tremendous blessing of spending special moments with Kai.

He is now an angel shining brightly, and for such a little soul, he had touched the lives of so many.

In his little casket, he was wearing my wristband that I gave him. I know that, regardless of the challenges that I have faced and continue to face, there's been a little boy in this world to whom I have made a difference.

I think that making a difference to others is what life is all about. Life is about waking up every single day, knowing in our hearts that we can make a difference in someone else's life.

Every day, we are in a position to help people to live their dreams, to shape their futures, and, above all else, give of ourselves, without expecting anything in return.

TIME & HEALTH ARE
TWO PRECIOUS ASSETS
THAT WE NEITHER
RECOGNISE NOR
APPRECIATE UNTIL THEY
HAVE BEEN DEPLETED.

EMBRACE YOURS NOW &

LOVE EVERY
MOMENT.

① BEFORE I WAS BORN

It was 1983. My mother, Kerri, went to the doctor because there were to be no more kids; my parents had decided that three crazy daughters were enough. The plan was to have her tubes tied. When she got in there, the doctor said, 'Either congratulations or commiserations.'

Mum thought maybe there was a problem with her health, but when he said he could probably help her out in six months, she knew she was pregnant. Mum was terrified by the prospect of another child, but Dad always wanted a boy.

In fact, he had already named the first, second, and third child Michael, but as he apparently used to say, he missed having a boy each time by half an inch.

My mum and I at 6 months old, naive to what was growing inside.

My family lived in the beautiful country town of Crossmaglen, which is 15 minutes south-west of Coffs Harbour on the east coast of Australia. We lived on a 5-acre property with fruit trees, chickens, dogs, a massive vegetable garden and a few sheep. It was a very tight-knit community where everyone knew everyone. People were accustomed to helping each other.

Neighbours routinely swapped food and other goods. My mum called it God's Country. We had properties all around us, most of which were banana plantations. We had a family living behind us who grew 10 acres of bananas. My mum told me that due to a lack of rain at the time, our neighbours sprayed their bananas to get them ready to be sold. Mum discovered much later that before our neighbour made the aerial spray, he had asked his wife to leave the house because it was suspected that she was pregnant.

At this stage, Mum was seven months pregnant. The very next day after the bananas were sprayed, she went into an early labour. Fortunately, the medical staff were able to stop the premature labour, and Mum went on to have a full-term pregnancy. To this day, we believe that it was the spray that caused her to go into labour, and we also suspect that it was the cause of many other health challenges.

On 2 May 1984, Mum had a painless delivery. She said that she was certainly aware that she was in labour with the girls, but she had no idea that she was in labour with me.

During the delivery, a physician by the name of Dr Scott was our gynaecologist. He waited for Mum to experience signs of labour pain, which never arrived, although she was trying to push.

She started to push, and my head was partly out when the doctor noticed that the umbilical cord was wrapped around my throat. He asked Mum to stop pushing, and any woman who has ever given birth will understand that's almost impossible to do at that stage in labour. What Dr Scott and Dad experienced was something they both described as a miracle.

The doctor pushed my head back in and somehow I twisted around, the cord came loose, and out I came. As Dr Scott held me up in the air, he said: 'This child is here for a reason.'

My family and extended family were so delighted to add another member to the Crossland household. Dad finally had his son and Mum finally did what needed to be done to ensure there were no more surprises — four children were more than enough.

Life on the farm was ideal — so green, so fresh and so quiet.

We had a beautiful little freshwater creek that gently flowed through the back part of the property, and we would always swim there and play as a family.

These good times on the farm with my family were more complicated than I remember, though, because of the dark cloud of fear, heartache and pain that would consume us all for many long years. As we grow older, we tend to forget about the wonderful moments we shared together as a family, and instead reflect only on the challenging times. As adults, I think many of us forget to have a good time and to simply enjoy life.

Instead, we get stuck in a rut of trying to be mature and grown-up, until the rare times that we take a moment to look back. It is then that we realise that we are now much older. We have missed much of the excitement of what life is all about.

The good times on the farm with my family were about to come to an end, as a dark cloud of fear, heartache and pain was about to take over and consume us all for many long years.

THE STRONGEST PEOPLE

AREN'T ALWAYS THE PEOPLE WHO WIN

BUT THE PEOPLE WHO

DON'T GIVE UP

WHEN THEY LOSE.

②

SUCH AN INNOCENT DAY THAT CHANGED OUR LIVES FOREVER

I was perfectly healthy, and by all accounts, I was considered a 'normal' baby; I ate plenty of food, and I was an active and happy little boy. Mum took me to the baby clinic regularly.

At the age of six months, the medical staff noticed that the growth of my stomach was a little too rapid for my age, but it was not discussed any further at that stage. Mum commented years later that the clinic nurses had simply said that maybe I was just over-indulging, because Mum was still feeding me as well as giving me solid foods.

There were no other symptoms, problems or sickness, so they just didn't give it another thought. Months later,

Mum took me to the doctor with my sister, because my sister had an ear infection. It was that day that our lives were turned upside down, and our entire lives changed forever. My sister Renee was born premature. Consequently, she suffered from a lot of ear, nose and throat problems in her earlier years. So, my parents took Renee to see our doctor quite regularly, and we were there for another check-up on her ears.

While I was there, Dr Scott made the comment that he was finally seeing me, because even though he delivered me, he hadn't seen me for 10 months. I was a happy, healthy baby, and had not been sick to warrant a visit. While at the surgery, Mum allowed me to crawl around the floor of the consultation room, and when the doctor picked me up to give me a hug, he noticed the size of my stomach. He made a comment about it, and in reply, Mum explained to him what the health clinic had said.

After he finished examining Renee, Dr Scott said he wanted to have a look at my stomach. He wanted to feel it to see whether there was anything there. Mum insisted that we needed to go home, because she had a routine with the three girls and me. It was 5.30 in the afternoon. After he felt my stomach, he arranged an immediate ultrasound.

So, we went for an ultrasound at a quarter to six that night. After several doctors looked at the results, they told Mum that Dr Scott was waiting in his surgery for us to return. That's when it began. Mum said: 'There's no way possible that Dr Scott would still be there at 6.30, because he would have gone home. We have to go home.' But he was there waiting.

He didn't give us any information about what it was, although he said to Mum that it could possibly be a large build-up of fatty tissue in my stomach. He also said we had to be in Sydney the following day. I guess that was the exact moment when our lives, and the lives of everyone else who was a part of our family's lives, changed forever.

After all, it was just the six of us who lived out on the farm at Crossmaglen. Then, without warning, Mum and I were ripped away from the family for many years to come. Mum and I arrived in Sydney, with everyone praying that it was a benign lump in my stomach.

Then Dr Mary Bergin came into our lives, and at that stage, the family had no idea she would be a part of it for so many years. She asked Mum whether she knew anything at all about childhood cancer.

Mum's first words were apparently: 'Kids don't get cancer.' Mum and many of our family members and friends honestly believed that cancer was something you got when you got old.

Dr Mary then broke the news to Mum: it was likely that I had cancer. Nevertheless, there were a lot more tests and scans that had to be done before the diagnosis could be confirmed. Mum said that her immediate thought was: 'It's not true; it just can't be, because kids don't get cancer.' Late that afternoon, the diagnosis was confirmed.

To this day, Mum says that it was like time stood still, and the words came out in slow motion. Pain filled my mum's heart when she heard: 'We have found a mass in his stomach; your son has neuroblastoma Stage 4 of the central nervous system. It is the size of a football, and there are several more throughout his abdominal area. There's just too much. I am sorry, Kerri, his survival rate would be no more than 4 per cent; we can't help him.'

What do you do when you're told that it's all over? You can roll over and die, or you can fight to the very end. 'There's nothing we can do,' they said. In a nutshell, this meant: 'Go home with a 96 per cent chance of death.' But in life it's not your adversity that defines you; it's how you deal with it.

As you may have already gathered, one of my favourite proverbs is 'I cried when I didn't get a new pair of shoes until I saw a boy who had no feet.' To me, this is a tremendously powerful way of saying that we need to compare our challenges and adversities with those of others in order for us to realise how lucky we truly are.

As a baby my life was 96 per cent hopeless, but there was still 4 per cent hope, and come hell or high water my mum was going to see to it that we never quit. We would be among the 4 per cent who survived.

It was not until we were taken downstairs to the oncology ward that reality hit. Years later, Mum commented that when we walked in there, it was the darkest place she had ever entered. Inside the ward, there were kids everywhere with no hair, needles up their noses, and parents who were completely heartbroken.

With the help of the hospital staff, we found our room and settled in for what was going to be a very long road. Mum felt so alone; she was so isolated, lost and truly scared of what each day was going to bring. We just needed some hope. Hope is one of the most powerful words in the dictionary, and if we could just get a little taste of hope, then that might be all that was needed to fight a good fight in order to win.

More than anything else, my parents hoped that the doctors would actually treat me. Instead, they did more and more tests and continued to say: 'We are sorry, but there is just no treatment that would save your son.' We couldn't just go home. Mum repeatedly asked whether there was any possibility that the doctors could treat me.

'Surely, there's got to be something!'

They relentlessly replied, 'No.' This went on for four days, however for Mum this would have felt like a lifetime. The phone calls to the family back home were heartbreaking. Dad did not know whether to tell my sisters and the rest of the family that I was dying, or to continue to hope and pray.

Today, I try to put myself in my parents' shoes and to imagine how they dealt with this type of fear and pain. I have come to the conclusion that you can simply never understand until you walk in the same shoes. I pray that I never walk in those shoes.

Dr Mary came in to see me and my mum on the fifth day of my hospitalisation. She said they had two American doctors visiting the hospital. She was going to put my case to them. 'Still there is no hope, so don't get carried away.'

So, my mum waited and waited with me for three hours, which, she has said many times since, felt more like three weeks. Mum's heart was racing and tears flowed freely down her face, but she said she constantly tried to hide it from me as she didn't want me to see that she was upset. Then, slowly, the door opened.

Dr Mary came through the door with an emotionally detached look on her face: 'Kerri, they're prepared to have a look and try, but they promise nothing.' Mum cried out loud, as if they had found a cure, purely because our hearts finally had a little hope in them. Mum hugged me so tight and didn't want to let me go.

I think there are plenty of times in people's lives where they're faced with a challenge where they just want to quit. They just want to walk away. They think it's too hard. It goes without saying that I'm so grateful every day that Mum didn't quit on me. Mum's outlook on life, her courage and optimism has, no doubt, continued to shape me and many others throughout my journey.

Obviously, there was still a lot of fear and worry for my family, because I was so sick. Mum believes, as a parent, you would do everything and give your utmost for your children, whether it is treating them for a common cold or a broken arm. She believes that any parent would stand by their child no matter how dire the situation, and do everything in their power to get their children through their battles.

It was a massive sacrifice for Mum to be away from my three sisters and our Dad for such long periods of time in hope that the treatment worked.

We were a seven-hour drive from our hometown, and with very minimal money, there was no way that we could afford regular visits or even trips home when my white cell count was up.

EVERY DAY
HOLDS THE POSSIBILITY OF A MIRACLE.

 KEEP STRIVING! IT MIGHT BE BEHIND THE VERY NEXT DOOR.

(3) TREATMENT

When the doctors suggested they'd start the treatment, Mum said they provided her with a summary of what the treatment would involve. Again, there were more tears and mounting fears within the family. Mum poorly understood the chemotherapy and doctor speech, but years later she said she was just happy they were going to try to save me.

The medical staff apparently kept reminding Mum that the odds of my survival were extremely low. The family didn't really take that news into consideration. Instead, they merely thought: 'Treatments are starting, so we've got hope.'

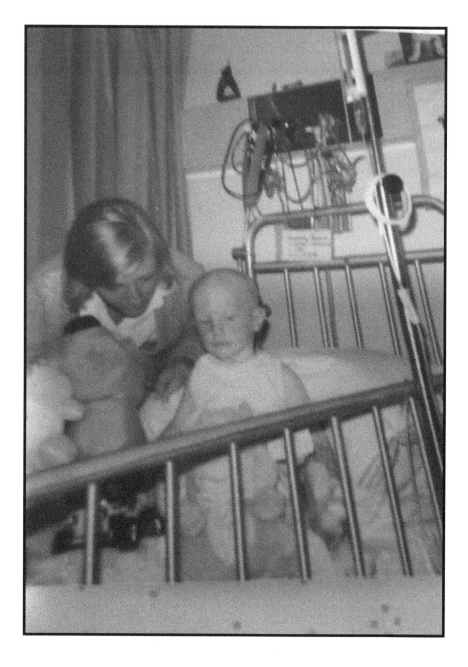

Mum and I on my first birthday, about to receive my first dose of chemotherapy at Camperdown Children's Hospital.

The doctors came in to inform Mum that they were going to start me on my treatment: 'They'll be starting in the morning.' It would be 2 May, the very first anniversary of my birth — I was barely a year old. Mum remembers asking the medical staff whether we could hold off for just one day so that I could enjoy my special day with my family, but their reply was as definite as it was immediate: 'Every minute counts.'

Rather than focusing on the grim facts and the excruciating side-effects that the treatments would have on my tiny body, my family later explained to me that they had decided to see the first day of my treatment as marking the time that we started to beat this cruel and insidious disease.

As Mum told me when I was old older, a cake arrived the very next morning, bearing one little candle. Nevertheless, it was a very short-lived celebration; one moment, the candle was blown out, and the next, one of the doctors marched through the door, followed by some of the nurses. It was time to commence round one of chemotherapy treatment, which provided my best hope of survival. My family really had no idea whatsoever how it was going to make me feel, or the impact that it was going to have on my body.

On the first day of my treatment, the doctor located my strongest vein, and through it the first lot of chemotherapy was injected. Years later, Mum told me that her immediate reaction was a feeling of excitement, but her belief that this was the stuff that was going to both rapidly and very effectively make me better turned out to be very short-lived.

Within five minutes, I started projectile vomiting, and the vomiting could not be stopped. It was as violent as it was persistent. In fact, according to Mum, the vomiting was so intense that the back of my throat became so badly burned it would bleed. Then, after the vomiting stopped, I could not eat, because the burns turned into painful and tender blisters. At the start of my treatment, my cycle was nine days on and three days off, and after every treatment, Mum became more convinced that I was going to die. I was just so sick.

Years later, Mum told me that for a while she started to leave the room during the treatment — just so that she could sit outside to get some fresh air. While outside, she would cry so hard, because she was just so helpless; there was just absolutely nothing she could do to either make me better or ease my immense suffering. I recall that as I grew older, my mum would always try to hide her tears from me, because she would never want me to see her visibly upset.

Regardless of her efforts to hide her sadness from me, as a one-year-old I would have been intuitively aware of when she was sad. Her eyes were constantly glassy, even though she worked so hard to hide her fear and sadness from me. Her unflagging and selfless strength is something that I will forever admire. To this day, her strength instils in me both inspiration and a determination to be like her.

A number of years after treatment, Mum explained she'd very quickly realised my first round of treatment was not going to equate to a short or temporary hospital visit, because the side-effects of the treatment were taking a serious toll on my body. In fact, she recalled one morning she awoke from sleeping in the chair beside my bed, only to see a look of despair, confusion and fear on my face. I was sitting up in bed, holding handfuls of my own hair, and trying to comprehend what was going on.

Throughout the night, my eyelashes and eyebrows had fallen out, and I was starting to look like a gravely ill little boy — much like a number of other children in the ward who had undergone the same treatment and died.

After a year had passed, Mum came to a level of acceptance about where we were headed within the hospital environment, and the journey we had no choice but to take. She was remarkable. She could always see the light and she constantly managed to maintain her optimism and hope, irrespective of how low and dark our days became during the treatment journey.

Even as a little guy, I apparently always loved to help others. Mum tells stories about what she used to do after I had my chemotherapy; she would try really hard to get me to sleep, because when I went to sleep after chemotherapy, I would not vomit. At two and a half years old, I began to tell the other children in the ward to do exactly the same thing as my mum kept trying to do for me.

The other children were in their beds, awake, vomiting, and extremely sick and miserable. According to Mum, I would stand up in my cot and instruct the other children: 'Hey, boy; you go to sleep. You won't be sick.' Clearly, I was keen to share with the other kids in the ward what had helped me.

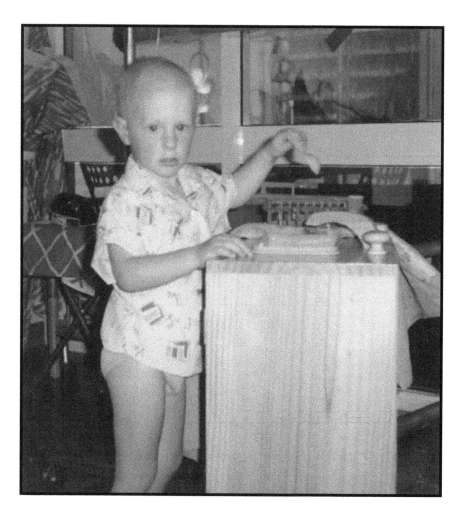

Me at 18 months old, having chemotherapy through a drip into my head so I can have two hands to play with.

On my own, I also worked out that if I counted to one hundred, the needles would be in and the pain in my hand would be gone before I even knew it, so I got very good at counting, and boy, did I learn fast!

After the chemo had really started to kick in, my mum started carrying me around, like most mothers do. One morning, I just started crying incessantly, and Mum could not understand why. The crying continued for two days, and my mum said to the doctor: 'This is not normal; please do something!'

Dr Mary ran heaps of tests and found that the drugs had made my bones so brittle that they had cracked. I had several fractures under my armpits, around my elbows and both knees. This was caused by one of the drugs, called vincristine. They stopped the drug immediately and I had to wear a helmet. I was in a cast, and elbow pads and knee pads had to be worn to prevent further damage! It was critical that we protected my bones as the pain was immense.

This went on for two months, and finally, the bones repaired themselves. Unfortunately, Dr Mary needed to restart the vincristine again. I can only imagine the pain Mum would have felt being so utterly helpless, and not being able to help or take my pain away.

There were times during the days of chemotherapy treatment that I was not permitted by the medical staff to be outside in the sunlight. Sometimes, there would be around 15 to 20 kids outside playing baseball, and for once, these kids were actually enjoying their lives. All of the parents had a ball, and we had to run around the yard, still attached to the trolleys that held our intravenous fluids, which in many cases had become permanently fixed to our hands.

Dr Mary would come out to yell at Mum. She'd say: 'It's wonderful what you're doing, but Michael's the only child that shouldn't be out there.' Mum never wanted to treat me any differently from all of the other kids. For instance, from a young age, she insisted that I use the toilet in the hospital. She taught me how to make my bed, as well as how to use a knife and fork. Ultimately, she made me feel like I was a normal kid — at least I thought so anyway.

Throughout the treatment journey, Mum continued to remain very naive about blood groups, and she also had a poor understanding of the damage that the chemotherapy was doing to my normal bodily functions. On one occasion, it was getting really close to Christmas. Mum just so desperately wanted to go home to be with Dad and the girls so that the family could spend Christmas together.

Regardless, Dr Mary informed my mum that my bloods were not good, and that we couldn't go home; we had to stay where we were during the Christmas holidays. I remember that Mum felt so strongly she ended up getting a bit nasty with the doctor, and she accused Dr Mary of being inhumane.

She even went as far as criticising Dr Mary for having no consideration for our family. Even at three years old, I felt that Mum's complaints against Dr Mary were very unfair.

Dr Mary basically acted like an old-school teacher, and she firmly and authoritatively requested for Mum to venture outside my room into the hall, so that she was away from me.

My mum obediently followed her request, which sounded more like an order, and Dr Mary followed her into the hall. Even though they were in the hall, I could still hear their conversation.

As a child, I thought the first question Dr Mary posed to Mum was really weird: 'How old do you think I am?' Years later, Mum said that she had actually tried to be very kind in her answer to the doctor.

She replied, 'Strange question, Mary. Around 45?' Mum said she looked much older than that, but she was trying to be really nice, hoping that the doctor would be flattered by Mum's response and would let us go home to the rest of our family for Christmas.

Dr Mary sounded weary, although nonchalant about the answer my mum had given: 'I've just turned 39.' Dr Mary had white-grey hair that was pulled back severely into a little ponytail; I suppose it was her hair that made her look older than she really was, but as a kid, it was hard to tell. I mean, when I was a child, anyone over the age of 15 seemed 'old' to me.

She continued to address my mum: 'I just want you to know something ... your three daughters? I don't give a damn. Your husband? I honestly don't give a damn about him either. As far as your son is concerned, we are going to do absolutely everything in our power to keep him alive.' Mum just sat there, and for once, she had absolutely nothing to say.

I mean, what does a person say after being served an impressive and irrefutable blow like that? Mum just sat there, and years later, she told me that while she was sitting there, she repeated the following inside her head, like a mantra: 'From now on, it will be: Yes, sir. No, sir. Three bags full, sir.' Dr Mary was extraordinary.

She certainly had the courage to stand up and fight when others had not wanted to fight for me at all. She was just like Mum; she never quit, and she never let go. Ever.

In our time in hospital, we came to meet some delightful families, many of whom I still remember. There was one lady in particular who warrants a special mention. Her name was Ingrid, and she was Dutch. Her son, Mitchell, had a Wilms tumour. As it turned out, he had his kidney removed on the first day that I started chemotherapy.

As you may recall, I would projectile vomit while receiving chemotherapy, and Mum was stricken by what she was seeing.

Mum later told me that one day while I was getting treated, Ingrid simply just appeared out of nowhere behind Mum, and she said to her: 'Hello; my name is Ingrid.' Mum looked up at Ingrid, and Ingrid continued to address my mum, in front of me and the staff who were administering my treatment: 'I know what you're going through. There's not much we can do.

How about you and I just go outside? We'll sit down at the tree for five minutes. Then, we will come back, because there's nothing we can do.'

The nursing staff agreed with Ingrid's suggestion as well as her rationale. They said to Mum, 'Maybe you really should go outside for a while', because Mum was very distressed by my screaming and by how violently ill the treatment was making me.

So, apparently after a bit more convincing from Ingrid, they retreated outside together to sit under a tree. It was really hard on Mum, but the louder I cried, the louder Ingrid spoke. The more Mum announced 'I've got to go inside', the more Ingrid insisted: 'No, you don't. Until they are finished administering the chemotherapy, we will remain sitting outside.' From that moment on, Ingrid and Mum became the best of friends, and Ingrid was just a pillar of strength for our entire family. Sometimes in life, we simply need to draw a line down the middle of a page. On the left-hand side, we write down the things that are within our control. On the right-hand side, we write the things that are out of our control. Too often, we spend so much energy focusing on the items that belong on the right-hand side of that page, futilely trying to fix the things that are completely out of our control.

Nonetheless, during the phase of our lives when I was being treated for childhood cancer, more than anything, we really needed to muster all of our energy, our strength, and all of our courage, so that we could begin to focus on the things that were both within our control, and that required our attention. Had we continued to focus on the things over which we had no control whatsoever, neither of us would have coped at all.

Mum rarely left my side. She would be there when I woke each day, and she was always holding my hand when I drifted off to sleep every night.

Due to the volume of tumours I had, the treatment plan was to maintain a shrinkage program for as long as my body would allow it. One unfortunate attribute of neuroblastoma, which is the type of tumours that I had, is that the tumour has a tendency to build a membrane around itself.

Consequently, it can become resistant to chemotherapy. Most unfortunately, by the time I was around two and a half, my tumours' resistance to the chemotherapy had slowly become apparent to the medical staff, and, more gradually, to my family. This realisation certainly had the impact of raising the fear and distress of my family to unprecedented levels.

There was simply no other choice, the doctors explained: 'We have to operate now, because the chemotherapy is not working. Sadly, Kerri, if we don't get it all in surgery, it will be over, and the chances of him coming out of surgery are not great.' When they got me prepped for surgery, Dr Mary came into the room.

They had me on the trolley, all ready to go, and Mary gave an instruction to the wardsman: 'Let the mother carry him.' Mum looked at her, and Dr Mary explained: 'It could be the last time, Kerri.' I can only imagine the overwhelming pain, the terror, and the uncontrolled, raw mixture of emotions that Mum experienced as she carried me into the white room where they were going to cut me open, kissing me for possibly the very last time.

I remember that she was desperately trying to show no emotion at all; it brings tears to my eyes as I type these memories and recall these events. Her devastation and fear had to have been profound, and yet, as always, she kept her emotions in check for my sake.

Prior to my operation, my mum and dad had their blood checked to ascertain their blood group. Dad's blood was found to be compatible with mine, so he asked the doctors whether he could possibly donate some of his blood to me. He'd get off the beer. He wouldn't consume anything unhealthy at all, so his blood would be of optimal quality for his son's needs.

The medical staff insisted that it wasn't necessary. Still, Mum and Dad started to become a bit insistent about Dad donating his blood to help me. They wanted to do it, because the HIV virus was poorly understood at that stage, and it was widely believed to be rampant and easily contractable at that time. They wanted to cover all bases. Again, the medical staff insisted to my parents that using Dad's blood to replace my own during the surgery was absolutely unnecessary.

Six hours was the amount of time that the operation took, and Mum waited and waited, constantly praying that everything was going to be OK, that her little boy was going to come out alive, and that the doctors would come out of surgery to deliver her the news that she so longed to hear: that the surgery had gone like a dream, the tumours had all been removed, there had been no complications, and that ultimately, her little boy would be OK.

Unfortunately, when one of the doctors finally left the theatre to report to my mum about how the surgery had gone, she did not get what she had prayed for at all. In fact, they said exactly what she feared the most. 'Kerri, he is still alive, but only just. We lost him for nearly two minutes, but he is hanging in there.

However, we are sorry, but we didn't get it all, and there is simply nothing more that we can do. Unfortunately, Michael had a very bad bleed through the surgery; he had two bags of blood, which at the time, we weren't concerned about.

However, we have been notified that, unfortunately, the blood that we did give him through surgery wasn't screened. Now, we have to undertake five years of HIV screening to ensure that he has not contracted the virus.'

Years later, my mum said that this day was the day she became broken; not only was she a broken mother, but as of that moment, she had a broken spirit and a lost soul. She could scarcely believe the words that the doctor had just said, but remarkably, somehow, she did not lose hope. She said that the first thing that I said when I came out of surgery was that I wanted an ice block, and that I wanted to play ball.

My family were flown down to Sydney so that they could spend my last few moments with me.

After I came out of surgery, I told my mum that I went to God's house. Mum tried to convince me that my mind was just playing tricks on me, because of all the flying that I had done, heading back and forth from Sydney to Coffs Harbour. Mum reminded me years later that I told her I was only there for a couple of minutes, sitting on God's lap, looking down on the planes, the hospital, and me in the room.

I said it was so beautiful, that I was so healthy, and so free. God said to me: 'Your time is not now, my son. You have a big journey ahead of you.' My mum recalled the surgeon told her I had died on the operating table for nearly two minutes.

She cried in front of me, and she later told me that she felt as though all of her prayers had actually been answered.

The weight, the fear and the worry had been taken from her almost instantaneously, and she felt as though she could breathe again for the first time in a very long time.

I regularly look around myself, and I witness people getting angry and frustrated because of First World problems: there's traffic on the road, or because they are asked to pay six dollars for a bottle of water in a five-star hotel, or it's too hot or too cold.

Every day, every single one of us, regardless of how optimistic or positive we are, complain about trivial, inconsequential and non-life-threatening problems.

It makes me think, 'Geez! If only these people were to face real problems and real heartache, would it still be a massive concern for them?' I think that it's so important that we don't wait for the phone call that changes our life, the doctor's visit that fills our hearts with fear, that once-in-a-lifetime decision, or an opportunity that changes everything.

We need to appreciate the finer things in life, love our challenges, grow from the hurdles that we face, and learn every day from every mistake we make.

4

ANOTHER GLIMPSE OF HOPE

My family was told I was going to be dead within four weeks, but just three days after the doctor had made this announcement, another doctor came into my room. He said to my mum, 'Kerri, we have a test drug. We're going to try it on 25 kids. We've got 24 candidates. We want to give your son the opportunity of a future.'

I truly believe that hope is one of the most powerful words in the English dictionary. If you can instil hope in somebody's life, you can instil determination, courage and passion, which can allow you to overcome anything.

I started this test drug at 9.00 am on a Tuesday morning. It made all of us kids who were given the drug violently sick; it felt as though my insides were on fire, and none of the kids who were given the treatment were spared from this horrendous side-effect. Within 24 hours, the burning was so severe that we were all transferred from the oncology ward to the burns unit.

The side-effects of this drug were so grievous that we were all covered from head to toe in blisters. The nurses would wrap us up in bandages and lay us in baths full of ice to try to control our temperatures and to prevent our brains from frying. We would just lie there and cry; there was really nothing else we could do. The families who were watching their children go through the most agonising pain must have felt unimaginably helpless.

Within five days, one of the little boys in my room who was also receiving the treatment tragically passed away. My mum started to get very scared; she was so terrified of losing me that she could no longer hide her tears. I could see pure, unadulterated fear in her eyes when two more kids passed away from the treatment over the next 48 hours. Within just one month, 20 out of the 25 patients were dead.

I can only imagine what it must be like as a mother or a father to be forced to make the decision as to whether to inject the very drug that has killed so many other little children into their own child. Mum said that the hardest part about that journey was watching the tiny body bags that held deceased little children who had died from the same drug I was on, being wheeled out of the very room I had shared with them.

Within the second month of the treatment, the drug began to burn my internal organs, and I had sustained severe burns to my left lung. My liver and my kidney were also being destroyed, while the muscles around my heart began to deteriorate. By the third month of being administered the drug, I was the only one left in the big room that had once been filled with 24 other families. Within 90 days, 24 out of the 25 were dead. My mum was faced with an impossible decision: she could either decide to continue the treatment, which meant the decision to continue to burn me, with a very real possibility of having the same fate as the other kids who had died, or alternatively, stop the treatment, with the guarantee that I would die.

Constantly seeing the other kids leave the room, one by one, and not return, really escalated Mum's fears. At that stage, she started to direct her thoughts, feelings and communications towards cancer survivors. I think that was what gave her hope; she had to draw on the strength that these survivors gave her in order to instil true hope in her own heart. The tragedy of witnessing the deaths of so many other children was incredibly hard to deal with. You'd see them one week, and then the following week they'd be gone.

There was a little boy who had Stage 2 neuroblastoma who wasn't in my trial. We had seen him only two weeks prior to the day that he had finally gone home. Mum had tried really hard to connect with and relate to this family, because for far too long, she had only dreamed of one day taking me home.

Then one day, that same little boy was lying on the floor back in the hospital. Mum said to his mum, 'Why are you back? It looks like he has the mumps.' Unfortunately, he had suffered a massive relapse. As it turned out, he had over 30 tumours growing out of his body, and two days later, he was dead. That day was the day Mum took herself to St Mary's Cathedral. She went to a healing service with the intention of casting all of her burdens to the Lord to lighten the load. Mum says her first thoughts were, 'This one's too heavy for anyone to carry.' Still, she said she managed to hand it all over. She replaced her fear with faith, and years later, she commented that the strength she gained from that experience truly got her through. It was on the day of her visit to St Mary's Cathedral that she began to realise she was not alone, and the darkest and heaviest days were the days she was being carried.

Every single day, I know in my heart that I've had a much easier life than my mum. The only thing I had to contend with is the pain. On the other hand, my mum had to helplessly watch her tiny son in pain, while remaining absolutely helpless — and not only that, she had to make impossible decisions about my treatment. I cry every time I think of how it must have been for her. This realisation is what has always prevented me from sitting around and feeling sorry for myself. Instead, it has only spurred me on to keep fighting, to strive for greatness, and to absolutely never give up.

Life was very hard to take at times. While in isolation, we were allowed no visitors. If Mum came in to see me, she had to wear a gown and a mask. She tried so hard not to cry in front of me. She used to walk outside and sit on the veranda to hide her tears, and I would constantly be calling out for her. I am sure most people agree that life just gets too hard sometimes, and during those times, the only thing we can manage to do is to hope that it gets a little easier. Well, thanks to one very special lady, it did! We got very close to a nurse by the name of Jo Gooch. She was an oncology nurse who was absolutely amazed by my mum's courage and by the battles that I continued to fight. Jo had a big soft spot for me, and when Mum was too emotional to be with me, Jo would step in.

We were living at Ronald McDonald House, which was a place that undoubtedly saved my family much heartache, not to mention astronomical expense. The Ronald McDonald House kept us together, because there would have been no way my parents could have afforded to rent an apartment near the hospital on the days I was allowed to leave for just a day or two.

Late one night, I came down with a massive fever. Mum had no idea how to deal with a temperature of 41 degrees Celsius in an adult, let alone a small child. So, she did what she was told to do. She laid me in a bath of ice on top of a towel with a fan over me. Nevertheless, it just wasn't working. For whatever bizarre reason, late on that very night, Jo decided to come up to the house to visit me. She walked in, took one look at me, and she immediately took over.

She grabbed me, gave Mum the car keys, and we drove to the oncology ward. Jo actually had me hanging out of the car window in a desperate attempt to get my temperature down. That's when the febrile fit started. I used to have severe fits when I got high temperatures.

Yet within five minutes of nurse Jo taking over, it was all under control. Mum and I bonded so powerfully with Jo that we ended up moving in with her. During the hard times, if Mum didn't quite understand what the doctors were saying, she could speak to Jo about anything, regardless of the time.

Jo had a knack for putting all the medical jargon into layman's terms so that Mum could understand what was happening to me. It was understanding what was happening that helped her to get through it. Once Mum knew what the doctors were doing, she could accept it and follow through with their instructions. I truly believe that Nurse Jo saved our lives; one time in particular was after I had surgery.

I had gone seven hours without passing urine. Not passing urine can be a bad sign, because, as the doctors told Mum, they had taken all of my organs out of my body and placed them all on a table during the surgery. The doctors removed as much of the cancer as they could, then they placed my organs back into my body (although I am sure it's far from as simple as it might sound). Sometimes when vital organs are removed, the bladder can get twisted, which can stop you from urinating.

This is what the nursing staff thought must have happened. Fortunately for me, this happened at midnight. Jo was on oncology night duty that night, and Mum rang her to explain what was going on. Jo came straight over to Intensive Care, and she asked the sister whether she had tried everything to make me urinate. Jo once again just took over.

She grabbed me, took me over to the sink, and she put my feet under the running water. She splashed water all over me, and then the water fountain began.

Jo now has two beautiful children, and Mum and I are very proud to be their godparents. Making us godparents just shows so beautifully and powerfully the impact that Jo had on our lives for such a long time. Even when I go down to Sydney to have tests as an adult, I always stay with her.

* * *

Mum tells me stories about how she would have to attend death counselling once per week for two hours in order to deal with what they thought was going to happen to her son. She tells me a story about how she was lying in bed with me one day when I was around three or four.

She was not allowed to touch me, because I was so badly burned. She said: 'I remember this day like it was yesterday, Michael. You were lying next to me and you whispered to me. You said: "Mommy, I had a dream. My dream is, when I grow up, I want to be normal like everybody else."'

I didn't tell my mum that I wanted to be a professional athlete. I didn't tell her that I wanted to be a fireman or a police officer. I just wanted to be normal, like everybody else. I wanted to appreciate the finer things in life everyone else took for granted, such as going to school and making friends.

My mum tells me that it broke her heart when she heard that, so she did something that the doctors told her not to do. She leaned down into the bed to pick me up, because she desperately wanted to hold her little boy. She tore the skin off of my hands. She ripped out all my needles. She tells me through free-flowing, unchecked tears that on that day, she had tried so hard to take my pain away, but to her horror, she caused me much more pain.

I truly believe in my life that everything has happened for a reason. I can't speak for anybody else, but I reflect on my challenges and I know that every time I've been knocked down, I've learned something important. Each time, I become stronger.

Each time, I become more determined. The needles could no longer go in my hand because my veins had started to 'hide'. So, they took the bandages off my head. They told my mum to leave, which made me cry. I cried just long enough for the veins to pop out, and then, they inserted the needle into my skull to continue the treatment.

I could have complained because I had a needle in my head or I could rejoice in the simple fact that, for the first time in years, I had two free hands. It's not the adversity in our life that defines who we are; it's how we deal with our adversity that determines whether we lead remarkable lives. Life is all about choices. Every day, we are faced with choices that can reshape our tomorrows, and every day we are bestowed with the wonderful gift of the opportunity to enjoy today.

The drugs continued to burn long after I stopped taking them. Lung infections continued for months and months. These infections just wouldn't go away. Then one day, I had a visit from the respiratory doctor. He asked Mum to go for a walk with him and she got some news. No matter what the news was, my mum would always return to my room with tears in her eyes and say: 'Everything will be OK, son.'

I never told her that I could see in her eyes she was not telling the truth, but I always hoped that one day I could return her favour: if I ever had to hear the doctor tell me that my health was bad, then I was going to tell Mum that everything was going to be OK. Years later, I learned that the doctor had told Mum they were considering placing me on a lung transplant list because of the damage caused by the chemotherapy and the test drug.

Not only was it damaging my lungs, but it was damaging my heart as well. Mum looked at it as another hurdle. Mum asked whether there was any way that she could personally help the situation. To Mum's surprise, they asked Mum to get me to blow up balloons, blow bubbles with the bubble blower, and skip.

We continued to do this day after day, and I continued to take the antibiotics and medicines that the doctors prescribed. Then a miracle happened. Six months later, there was no need for a transplant. Someone upstairs was watching.

DREAMS ARE LIFE'S PURPOSE.

(5)

DREAMS SAVE LIVES

After many months, the skin finally grew back on my hands. My parents were both avid baseball and softball players, so my mum bought me a velcro glove and a velcro ball to play catch with. She would sit at the end of my bed and lob the ball to me, and I'd catch it and throw the ball back.

She told me in later years that she would get farther and farther away until she'd be outside the hospital room; she'd be throwing the ball past the doctors and past the nurses, and I would give it my all to catch the ball. I recall thinking at the time that I was the best baseball player ever, because I never dropped the ball, although I realised when I got older that the velcro may have had something to do with it.

I'd be in my room with the needle in my head, diving out of my bed, making the catch and trying to fire it back to her, past the doctors and nurses. When I started to get a little stronger and healthier, I would practise my sliding nearly every day; I'd run up and down the hallway and she'd run next to me with my trolley, the needle still in my head, and I'd be sliding into the base of the beds where Mum had piled loads of pillows to stop the ball travelling further. I would try to be as normal as I could, because this had been my first dream.

I tried to enjoy the little things that I was allowed to experience every day, whether it was sneaking outside for some fresh air without the nurses knowing, which made me feel very naughty, or waking up early to feel the warmth of the sun beaming through the hospital windows. Every night, I would go to bed and pray so hard that one day I was going to be allowed to go home to be with my family.

The cleaner always seemed keen to come into my room to clean my floor at 4 am, which invariably woke me up. Once I was awake, I'd have nothing to do, so I would turn the TV on. Back in those days, the only television networks airing at that time of day were the ABC and another channel that played the major league baseball in the United States. After playing catch with my mum and watching major league baseball on TV, all of a sudden I had another dream.

This dream was bigger than ever before; more sacrifices were needed and many laughs would be had by the sort of people who only ever tell you what you can't do in life. The dream was to one day play baseball in America.

Thinking back, I'm glad that these were the only channels airing at that time, because I would hate to have turned on SBS at 4 in the morning. Who knows what my dream could have otherwise been? Ha ha!

I think that there is great wisdom in the expression 'Shoot for the moon. Even if you miss, you'll land among the stars.'

If you have a dream, then you have a passion, a burning desire to see your dream come true. While you work towards the realisation of your dream, time goes by without you even noticing. Work is something that you enjoy doing, and you forget the world around you. When you wake up in the morning, it does not matter whether it is a sunny or a rainy day. You see every new day as an opportunity to take you closer to your goal. What other people say or think about your dream becomes irrelevant.

You simply know that you're going in the right direction. Because you're inspired, you feel a constant flow of energy.

If you feel this way, you have defined your dream and maybe your destiny. The only other ingredient to fulfil your dream is persistence.

As we ride the planet around the sun, life can sometimes be hard and complicated. We dream of living better lives or achieving great goals. For many, the state of our present lives results from being born into difficult circumstances or surviving tragedies.

Nevertheless, no matter where we find ourselves, our lives are also a reflection of all the choices we've made along the way.

It's crazy that some of the most powerful and influential people on this planet have faced true adversity and suffering throughout their upbringing. Still, these people never use that as an excuse to fail; instead, they use their experiences to harness their burning desire to succeed.

I have witnessed too often people who are violent towards their partners or their children because their own parents behaved in the same manner when they were kids. I don't see that as an excuse for bad behaviour at all. Instead, sometimes your parents and other people of influence can actually set the behaviour that you should not follow. You actually learn from their mistakes and poor behaviour.

Yet we still hear about people who overcame impossible odds to achieve great things in life. There are often tales of being at the right place at the right time, a coincidence, or meeting the right person just when they needed to.

Did the lucky few who made it just so happen to find Aladdin's magic lamp that delivered these miracles? How do the rest of us get one of those?

In my opinion, we all have a magic lamp. It is our unshakeable commitment to achieve our dreams. No matter where we find ourselves, I believe that this commitment is always inside and waiting to be tapped.

I was committed and wanted to be the person who did the 10 per cent extra and then fell into the 1 per cent category of achieving what many believed to be the impossible dream.

THE
POWER OF
NEVER GIVING UP
_____
IS LIFE
CHANGING.

6

THE DAY THAT WAS NEVER TO HAPPEN

After we had lived at the hospital for many years, when I was five the doctor finally said to my mum the words that she prayed for, but never thought she would ever hear: 'Kerri, take your boy home.' The excitement and the emotions elicited by that simple statement were almost too much to handle; she let out an almighty cheer and the tears just flowed down her face as she squeezed me harder than I thought possible.

But 'Take your boy home' did not mark the end of the conversation. The doctor went on to say that due to the after-effects of all the drugs, I'd never go to school, I'd never play sport, I'd be a house-bound baby, and if I reached my teenage years, it'd be a miracle.

My mum's heart sank, but she didn't allow it to sink for long because my mum and my family had always believed in miracles. She thought that this was just going to be another hurdle to deal with.

They had told her years before that I wouldn't make it to two years old, so who were they to tell her I wouldn't make it to 12?

Too often, we allow others to dictate our lives, but my family has always believed in our hearts that no human being determines when your life is up; God is the one in control.

My mum wanted my first dream to come true, which was to be normal like everybody else. She wanted to allow me to enjoy the simple things in life that so many of us just take for granted. So on Monday morning, straight out of hospital, she let me go to school like everybody else.

I imagined how school was going to be. I'd walk through the school gates. Everyone would be nice to me. I was going to make great friends. I was going to be the class clown. I was going to be the teacher's pet. Everyone was going to like me. Instead, I walked through the school gates and the school bully was there.

I've been called every name under the sun, including cancer boy, burnsy, odds-defier, baldy. I would be lying if I said that I didn't care. Mum used to tell me to remind myself of the saying, 'Sticks and stones may break my bones, but names will never hurt me', but that's not true; names absolutely do hurt you.

My time at school was tough. Really tough. I had imagined how it was going to be, and I was so wrong. I just wanted people to like me and be my friend.

I knew from a very young age that I was never going to be normal. While all the other kids were out in the playground, I would sit in the classroom every recess and lunch on my nebuliser (a device that looked like a miniature spaceship that vaporised medicine so I could breathe it in) to give my lungs the strength to simply walk to the bus stop of an afternoon.

There were many lonely days at school ahead. I could easily complain that I was stuck inside a classroom feeling different, or I could be excited that I was not in hospital.

I think that it is so important in life that we realise that it's not our adversity that defines us, but rather, how we deal with it. I started to reflect on another saying my mum often repeated.

She would say to me after a rough day at school: 'Son, remember: what doesn't kill you only makes you stronger.'

She was right; my mum was always right. The names, the different way I looked, and the challenges I had faced didn't kill me, but boy did they make me stronger.

Even though there were so many dark days, I was never really alone; not only did I have my family, and God, who never left my side, there were also many different charities that supported me through thick and thin.

The charities that came into my life completely lifted me out of pain and adversity, and they led me to normality, joy and happiness. One day, a lovely couple by the name of Tom and Nancy Strickland came into our lives, and what an impact they had! They were an absolute godsend.

They came to the property one day. I was outside in the yard with Mum. They introduced themselves to me, and they asked whether it would be at all possible for them to take me to a camp. Mum thought she wouldn't let me leave her sight at any stage, so she immediately replied, 'No.' Nancy said, 'It's JUST one week a year; you deserve a break.' All Mum could say was, 'I don't want a break. I just need to be with him.'

They explained what Camp Quality was all about, using the words optimism and resilience. They explained that the supervision they had over kids on camp was incredible.

They described the purpose of Camp Quality, which is to create a better life for every child in Australia who is living with cancer. They explained that they are committed to delivering national programs that build resilience and optimistic behaviours in these kids.

They talked in-depth about the word optimism and the hard work they take on trying to spread positivity, hope and enthusiasm by the way they interact with other people.

They talked about how driven they are with regard to maintaining their integrity, and about how they encourage the development of trust through personal leadership. They said that they are always celebrating life, with every day being an adventure.

They went on to say that they pride themselves on their accountability, that they always accept responsibility for actions and results, and that they accept nothing but excellence from their teams, encouraging them to seek greatness in all that they do. So, Mum relented and let me go.

The first time I went to camp, Mum admits that she must have called every second hour to find out where I was and what I was doing. The camps continued every year, which was a massive thing for me and all of our family. It was the one week every year when Mum didn't have to worry about me.

Camp Quality's key motto is, 'Laughter is the best medicine', and that's so true because we can either choose to frown at a situation, or we could laugh at it. We laughed. It was a really good feeling. I feel very privileged to remain heavily involved with Camp Quality. I have gone from a camper to a companion, and I am now the National Ambassador. It's a real honour.

Another organisation that was a huge support to me and my family is the Cancer Council, whose vision is to achieve a cancer-free future for the Australian community. With their mission in mind, they work with the community to reduce the incidence and the impact of cancer.

Their values are all about making a real difference. They seek to yield a major, positive impact on the lives of all Australians.

They never stop seeking to improve and innovate what they do, and they are prepared to take risks to achieve breakthrough results. They are passionate about their mission, and they maintain a deep value of the community and each other. They show empathy and respect, and they value all.

The Cancer Council holds a very special day, called Daffodil Day, and this was something that my family and I were heavily involved with right at the beginning. The daffodil has been recognised internationally as the symbol of hope for people in our community who have been touched by cancer, either directly or indirectly.

The daffodil heralds the beginning of spring, the season of hope, and the new life that it brings. It also reminds us that there is life after a diagnosis of cancer.

A lady from the United States offered to support our regional areas by bringing the flowers to our township so that we could sell them to raise money. I would go with my bald little head and my Camp Quality shirt to sell these beautiful flowers. The first year we sold every single flower.

The support and the money we made were overwhelming. What we realised at the end of the day is that everybody just wanted us to take the flowers home and to accept their money. 'Give the flowers to your family,' they would say.

Mum said it made her feel like the Mayor of Coffs Harbour. It was amazing: people whom I had neither met nor seen before in my life were so caring and so giving; it continued to give us hope.

By this stage, I had been home for some time now, and my family was trying to get my life back to normal — or as normal as they could make it. I was about to celebrate my sixth birthday, and this was going to be the first birthday that I had ever celebrated at home, so you can imagine how excited I was.

Before we had left the hospital, the doctor had talked about my future and how it did not look bright. However, one thing that was emphasised to my mum was to ensure that my stress levels were kept to an absolute minimum, because stress exerts a major influence on whether or not cancer returns.

Mum thought that she would throw a surprise birthday party. I had come home from a day at the park after enjoying some quality family time, when Mum asked me whether I would mind going to the garage to grab the broom.

I made my way down to the garage, and I opened the roller door. To my immense surprise, people jumped out of nowhere from behind the door, yelling: 'Surprise! Happy Birthday!' I was so frightened that in front of all my family and friends, I soiled my underwear.

My mum immediately thought back to what the doctor said — 'Do not stress him out' — and she had just done exactly that.

She told me that I cried, although I think it was more with embarrassment than fear. After getting all cleaned up, I had a wonderful afternoon, and I enjoyed the best ice cream cake you have ever seen in your life.

Ah, the memories; I'm sure as I grow old, it will not be the last time I soil my pants.

APPRECIATE THE
SUNSHINE
ONCE YOU HAVE
WEATHERED THE
STORM.

⑦

HEART STOPPED
AT AGE 12!

Another tremendous challenge for me as a child was the transition between primary school and high school. I went to a primary school with a total population of just 28 children. The school was in our small country village in Crossmaglen. Everyone knew everybody, and we only had one teacher who taught the entire school.

I graduated year six, and I headed off to high school. I attended Toormina High, where the total population of students was over 1200. The school had basketball courts, football fields, libraries, a massive hall, and different subjects were taught in different areas of the school. The drastic change in culture was extremely overwhelming.

It was very challenging to venture into this massive school and to know nobody, besides my two older sisters who were still attending the school.

For the first month, I felt like a real loner; I would roam the hallways, walk out onto the football field, head past the basketballers, and even wander into the library, trying to find where I could fit in. Even the handball courts were so packed that I could barely get anybody's attention, let alone try to make a friend.

It was a really tough time. I had finally made some good, solid friends at my primary school, but they had all gone to a private high school. I was feeling very alone. I think when you get to that point in your life, you really stop seeing reality; you think people are saying things about you, but they're really not.

You even become a little bit paranoid, but I continued to remember that my life could be so much worse. So, I reminded myself that life had been so much tougher in the past, to just stay strong, and to do my best not to show any emotion, because one day things would get better. And things did get better in the most remarkable way.

It was week five of term one and I was walking through the hallway alone again when a young girl with Down syndrome decided to start chasing me. I freaked out and ran as fast as I could until one of the boys in my year grabbed me, told me to hide under the seat, and said that he would cover the seat with school bags.

So, as he suggested, I jumped under the seat, and he and a group of other boys all sat in front of the bags. The girl just ran straight past us. When the coast was clear, I popped out from underneath the seat and the boys all introduced themselves to me. We all had a chuckle, and 18 years later, I'm still friends with those boys.

I was finally enjoying the life that I always wanted and never thought possible. I was finally at home with my family, I was finally making friends, and I was starting to live life on my terms. I was finally getting to play sport and loving the game of baseball, because I wasn't just playing it in hospital anymore; I was playing it for real.

We had a few challenges along the way, until one day the fear really set in. We would go down to Sydney every three months for tests, which were extremely taxing on the body, not to mention the family's finances.

This trip was expected to be just like all the others; I had to have a bone and gallium scan, ultrasounds and CT scans. There were special diets and I had to fast for some of these tests. At one point on the plane, Mum got up to use the bathroom. The flight attendant was sitting there with me having a good old chat, and everything was fine.

When we got to the hospital, the radiologist started the first scan, and no sooner had they started the scan than they found a massive lump in my stomach. Obviously, everyone felt immense panic. Dr Mary got called over to radiology, and they said: 'It doesn't look good.' That was Mum's greatest fear; that it would come back.

They had mentioned to Mum often throughout my treatment in previous years that even if I survived, the chance of recurrence is very high. Mum kept saying, 'It can't be, Mary. It can't be; please say it's not true.'

Dr Mary replied, 'I can see it, Kerri. Has he eaten?'

Mum snapped back: 'No. He ate nothing.' Mum then said to me accusingly: 'Did you eat anything, Michael?'

I said: 'Your chewing gum on the plane, Mum; I ate it all up.'

That was the lump that everyone panicked about. It was a big wad of chewing gum in my stomach, bolted while Mum had been in the bathroom. I love my chewing gum. I still love my chewing gum. It is easy to laugh about it now, but my poor mum nearly had a meltdown.

On our way home from hospital, my uncle who lived in Sydney suggested that we catch up. He said, 'Let's all meet up at McDonald's. We'll have lunch.' When we got into McDonald's, there was a big picture on the wall of the actual Ronald McDonald House where we used to stay.

I was standing there, engrossed in the picture. The manager came up to us and said to me, 'That's an amazingly big house, isn't it?'

I replied, 'No.'

The gentleman said, 'What do you mean "no"?'

My reply was: 'That house makes me sick.' This poor guy had no idea what I was talking about.

Then my uncle said, 'Michael spends a lot of time at Ronald McDonald House.' He lifted my hat to show him my shiny, still-bald head.

The gentleman said, 'You know what? It's a privilege to know someone that stays at that house. Let me buy you all lunch.'

My impulsive response was: 'We don't love your burgers. They're awful, but we like your ice creams.' So, we all got an ice cream cone. Uncle Wayne wasn't happy. Ha ha.

* * *

I was still obsessed with baseball; while I was never the best player, I always tried my best, and it took me until my twelfth birthday for me to reach the level of representing my hometown of Coffs Harbour. We went away to the country championships where they selected the top 16 players to represent New South Wales, and I can't begin to tell you how excited I was to make that team.

However, one week before we were due to fly out to the national championships, I became very unwell, and I was taken to hospital. I was told by the doctors I had glandular fever, and while I was in hospital I managed to catch even more viruses due to my low immune system. Then, my entire world changed forever.

I had four doctors on my left and my mother holding my hand on my right, where she has always been, and I went to take a deep breath in. The pain in my chest is something that's almost impossible to describe: the agony, the suffering, the sharpness and the intensity of the pain was mind-blowing.

At the age of 12, I had suffered my first major heart attack and my life was never going to be the same. Mum was petrified. She was actually asked to leave the room. She said she was behind the curtain; there was no way she was leaving the room. She said she stayed beside me while they did what they had to do. I heard them say: 'Clear.'

That was when Mum realised that they were using those paddles on me. She burst out crying and thought to herself: 'Why? Not again. Please don't take him from me.' A short time passed, which Mum said felt like days, and she heard me talking with the doctors.

That was when they discovered how much heart damage I had sustained from the cancer treatments. Again, we didn't let that beat us.

I often say that I have a VIP card to hospitals. I never got a free coffee or a stamp on my hand, but they certainly all knew me and treated me well. The feeling of being helpless is something that registers in my heart and my mind when I hear about these situations, because I think it's a really powerful exercise to step out of your own shoes and look at life through someone else's eyes.

Throughout the really tough times it would have been so hard for my mum. It would have been so difficult having a big family, with Dad taking care of the girls, although it was difficult to have all of my sisters with me because my parents didn't really want them to understand the severity of what I was going through.

All they ever wanted was for me to come home. That was my therapy. I used to even say to the doctors: 'Let me go home, Doctor. I'll get better.' Nine times out of 10 I did.

I was in hospital for many months and missed so much school, but, my mum being who she is, she never allowed me to feel sorry for myself, and she never allowed me to fall behind. She would have teachers come in every second day with schoolwork to ensure that I didn't miss out on learning. I was fortunate that year to be dux of my class, so I didn't need to repeat that year.

When I was finally allowed to go home, the doctor said something that really challenged me. He told me that I would never play sport again and that I must be very careful about how hard I exercised as the strain on my body and my heart had been immense.

I love it when people tell me what I can't do, because it makes me work very hard to show them that I can. I'm never out to prove other people wrong, but I just enjoy working hard every day to prove myself right. 'Can't' is a word that shouldn't be a part of anyone's vocabulary.

I refuse to believe that things can't be done. Have you ever noticed that some people are sometimes a little too quick to tell you why something can't be achieved?

When someone mentions the word 'can't', it might be about embarking on a type of project you've never done before, creating a new product, launching into a new country, applying for a great new job or winning a battle that CAN'T be won.

'Can't' is a word used by people who are just projecting their own fears out into the world, by people who can't see past their present limitations, and by people who don't realise that given the right mentality, they, too, can begin manifesting their dreams at a rapid pace. It's much easier to make excuses not to do something big and overwhelming than to simply put one foot in front of the other to start chipping away at the not-so-glamorous work of making your dreams come true.

Why do people do that?

I think that people are just so scared of making a mistake. It's a fear of failure, and a fear of embarrassment. Maybe they're fearful of change. I think it's a completely normal and healthy human response to feel all of these things when stepping into the unknown and when taking risks. But if you recognise that this fear is just a passing emotion that doesn't necessarily have to chain you into not making any moves, then you might be able to set yourself free.

Miracles are just a shift in perception from fear to love. For some people, it's just safer to do nothing rather than try something new. They can maintain the status quo. They don't want to rock the boat. They're in their comfort zone. But, life only really begins at the end of your comfort zone. It's overwhelming to imagine what a different world we would be living in if everyone listened to those who said it can't be done.

It used to be thought that it was not humanly possible to run a mile in less than four minutes. Yet, Roger Bannister broke the four-minute barrier with a time of 3:59.4. Soaring through the air in a flying machine? Can't be done, said the sceptics, including the Wright brothers' own father, who scoffed at the idea, saying that they should leave flying to the birds. Going into space? Can't be done. 'Can't' is an ugly word. It should be banished from our thoughts. Mindset is everything.

By simply making some minor adjustments to how we think and by removing the negative thoughts we tell ourselves, which leave us ruled by fear, we can make great strides towards our desired result.

Anything is possible if you have a clear vision and are willing to do the work. I've never accepted that I can't accomplish what I set out to do. There's simply no room for 'can't' in my life.

Henry Ford's quote is so apt in capturing this point: 'Whether you think you can or think you can't — you are right.' Whenever I've been told that something is impossible or something simply can't be done I just smile, and deep down inside, I say to myself: 'Just watch me.'

HAVE A GOAL
EACH DAY TO

CREATE THE
KIND OF SELF

THAT YOU
WILL BE
HAPPY TO
LIVE WITH FOR THE
REST OF YOUR DAYS.

8

BLOOD, SWEAT
AND TEARS

I had created a dream and a vision — to play baseball in America — so I needed to get out of my comfort zone and go out into this world and make it happen.

It's amazing what can be achieved when you can imaginatively extend yourself beyond what previously seemed impossible. By going deeper, and in doing so, understanding yourself better, you create a better balance. The heart and soul are enhanced.

Then, you become more focused on the positive. Most people are focused on what they believe they 'can't' do, and not on what they 'can' do. Fear is the paralysis and usually the culprit that knocks you down and holds you down to make you quit; I was never going to quit. I was going to live my life on my terms and make it happen, not let it happen.

I kept playing baseball, even though I was told not to, but I played a little smarter. I made sure that I never overdid it. I made sure I always warmed up adequately. I made sure I always cooled down properly.

I wasn't the fastest, or the biggest or the strongest, but I knew the game inside and out. I love the game. I just wanted to get better. I wanted to always try a little harder than everybody else.

I always wanted to make sure that I did the 10 per cent extra every time my coach asked me to do something. I wanted to make sure that I did that little bit more to not merely catch up with the others, but to leapfrog ahead of them at one stage in my life. I really wanted to make sure that I consistently did the 10 per cent extra that allowed me to fall into the 1 per cent who manage to fulfil their dreams.

I remember there was one man who was around throughout my childhood; he was very involved with baseball on a local level, and he used to always tell me that I was far too small to play baseball, and that I would never make it in this game.

Little did he know, that was all the fuel I needed to doggedly pursue my dreams. It took me until the age of 15 to get myself to the level I needed to be to, once again, represent my town of Coffs Harbour. I played so well at a tournament that I was selected to play for the New South Wales state team.

As fortune had it, one afternoon after the tournament was finished, I got a tap on the shoulder by a man who would change my life forever. His name was John Murray (he went by JM). At that time, he was the head coach and tour manager of the Brisbane Expos touring baseball team. They went to the United States once per year for three weeks, and they travelled around the country and played 15 games of baseball.

He told me that the program was not just about taking amazing athletes to America; instead, it was far more forward-thinking than that.

The tour was based around what he referred to as 'the A Principle', which was an acronym for Attitude, Ability and Achievements. The key word was Attitude. The day that he told me that I was in the team was the day I realised that my dream was only just around the corner from coming true. The clincher was that it was very expensive. It was $5000.

My family have never had money, so it was going to be a big challenge for me to get there.

I always wanted to do things off my own bat. We had to train every weekend in Brisbane and there was no way that we could afford the flights up and back all the time. I would play Saturday morning in Coffs Harbour, and then I would get on the 4.30 pm Greyhound bus to Brisbane.

I would get to Brisbane at 12.30 am. John, my coach, would pick me up, and we'd go back to his house. I'd fall asleep for a few hours, then wake up in the morning, have breakfast and head to Redlands Baseball field.

We trained from 9 am until 5 pm, and then I would head back into the city. I'd have some dinner with him and he'd put me on the 8.30 pm bus home.

I would get to Coffs Harbour at 4.30 Monday mornings. My mum or dad would come down to pick me up from the highway and drive me back out to Crossmaglen.

I would then shower, have some breakfast, put my school clothes on, go to bed for an hour or so, and then get back up to walk the 1.2 kilometres to the end of the road to get the school bus back to school.

If ever I missed a Monday morning of school, I wasn't allowed to go to training the following week. That was the deal that my mum and dad had set with me. My studies were never going to be negatively affected by playing the game that I loved.

I never missed one weekend of training because I never missed a Monday morning of school. (Although Mum never realised that I may have spent a few Monday mornings in the sick bay to get some rest. Ha ha.)

I had to make sure that I came up with the bus money every week on my own, though. Not only did I have to raise the $5000 that I needed to get myself to the United States, but I also needed to raise the $80 per week to get on the bus.

I would do pretty much anything in hard labour to make that money. I would wash cars and weed driveways. I remember spending a lot of time with one of my coaches, Kerry Owen, who lived out at Crossmaglen.

I would mow his lawns, wash his cars, pick up palm fronds, and pick fruit for him. I would do whatever it took to make sure I got the $80 to get me on that bus so I could get out and learn, really hone my skills, and nurture the talent that God had given me, so I could continue to get better and compete.

I remember one day I was knocking on doors asking whether I could do some yard work to raise the money I needed, and I finally managed to get inside the door of a really rich couple. They had the most beautiful home and they had all the fancy cars.

They finally agreed that I could help them out around their home, so they asked me to weed their driveway, which must have been at least 100 metres long. It took me nearly eight hours, and I was exhausted after a huge day, bending at the hips to pull out weeds.

When it finally came to pay day, he said to me that I had done a fantastic job. He handed me an envelope and said, 'Thanks for your effort.' I could not wait to leave the property so I could rip open the envelope to see how much cash had been stuffed in there.

I ran down his driveway, and when I was out of sight, I stopped to open the envelope. Inside the envelope were two $5 notes. I had worked nearly eight hours and he had paid me $10. I couldn't believe it; I was thinking that I had probably made enough for at least one week's worth of bus trips. I felt momentarily angry, but after a little while, I laughed it off and thought: 'Only $70 to go.'

The $5000 to get me on that plane wasn't easy either. It was a hard slog. Raising that money meant lots of raffles, trivia nights, auctions and fundraising, but I managed to get there thanks to the generosity of the local community.

I must have knocked on the door of every single business in Coffs Harbour, saying, 'Please, can you donate something? Let me buy something off you at cost price, and try to either give it away in a raffle, or auction it off to get me over to America.'

The support that I received was unbelievable. I feel so privileged and blessed to have had them along as part of that journey. I guess it made that milestone of playing baseball in America that much more worthwhile because nothing was ever handed to me. It was hard work, determination, commitment, and the inner belief that I was going to get there that allowed me to achieve it.

Sadly, these days it's almost an expectation that people are handed everything for nothing, including not only what they need, but also everything they want. In my opinion, this instils a complete lack of appreciation for anything, and the hard work needed to achieve anything is just disregarded.

The auctions were done, the raffles were finished, and the fundraising was over. The grand total amount raised was $5530. I was over the moon, because I was going to America, and I had spending money.

My doctors were concerned about me flying for such lengthy periods of time because my immunity was still poor. I had to pack what looked like a lifetime supply of medication and vitamins, and I was ready to go. I was really focused on how hard I had trained and what I was eating, so that I could be as fit and as healthy as possible.

The weekend prior to departure we were given our uniforms; I cried when I received my jersey with my special number on the back. It had the name, CROSSLAND, with the number 24, in large, bold, black print.

Very few people that day realised why I was so emotional and why that number meant so much to me. You see, I never played by myself when I was wearing that number; I was always playing for the 24 little angels who did not make it through that horrible test drug.

John, my coach, told me that he knew why I was in tears, and he held me like I was his own son. He said that he was so proud of me and the determination that I had shown.

He asked me what I wanted to achieve while I was in America. I responded with a clear answer: 'I just want to turn a double play in the States.'

I realised at training that I was never going to be the biggest, the strongest, the guy that was going to be the starting shortstop, the superstar, or the guy on whom they relied to make sure that we could win or compete as effectively as we could. These guys were just giving me an opportunity, because I had a little bit of talent, a big heart and a massive dream.

The day had finally come when I had to say goodbye to my family, and then I was up and away. I think I packed four weeks early, because I was so excited. My mum cried — I think for many reasons.

It was not just that she was going to miss her boy. I think she was also reflecting on the past and thinking to herself: 'How has this happened? My little boy, who was not supposed to make his second birthday, is now a young man and he is heading to America to live his dreams.'

I think this point in my life was truly a defining moment. It proved to me and my family that anything is possible if you work hard and dream big. I remember flying into Los Angeles feeling exhausted but excited as I looked out the window and saw baseball fields everywhere, tall buildings, and eight-lane highways.

We got off the plane and headed through customs, wearing the biggest smiles on our faces. We headed outside to get on the bus, and we all looked the wrong way, because the cars came flying past us on the wrong side of the road!

I remember getting into the hotel room and needing to go to the toilet after all of the fantastic plane food. I finished doing my business and flushed the toilet; I was immediately frightened, because the toilet started filling up — the contents were getting closer to the top, rather than disappearing!

I yelled at my roommate, and he started laughing uproariously; he was a veteran traveller, so he knew exactly what was going on. The toilet eventually began to suck the water back, and its contents finally went down with it. It had me panicking for a moment there.

It was time for game one. We listened to our national anthem, the Australian flag was being raised, and as I ran out onto the baseball field, I heard my name announced through the PA: 'From Coffs Harbour, New South Wales, number 24, Michael Crossland.' I had goosebumps, and tears streamed down my face.

The sacrifices were worth it. The dedication and discipline were worth it.

The commitment had all been worth it, because I had achieved something that people told me all my life I would never ever be able to achieve. It was late in the game when I played second base.

My dream of turning a double play became a reality. It was the game-ending double play, and I had not realised that John had told the rest of the team about my dream.

They hoisted me onto their shoulders and allowed me to bask in my moment in the sunshine. I think that nothing is impossible when you want to fulfil a dream. Many people will tell you that

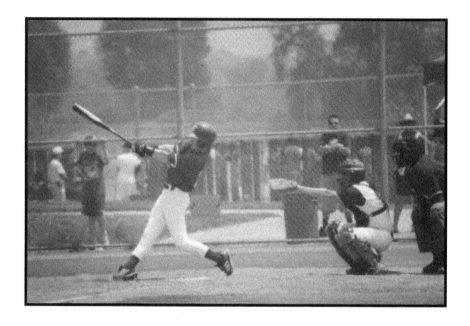

Me at 15 years old, hitting a double down the right field line playing baseball in Redlands, California.

you can't do it, and that you don't have what it takes, but if it is in your heart and you feel it, there is nothing that will stop you.

While there we were hosted by families in a town called Redlands. They were a beautiful community and some of the most amazing people that you could ever meet in your life.

The man who ran the American side of this baseball program was named Steve Chapman, and boy did we become life long friends! Through JM, they had found out a little of my story, and Steve had a list of people from the community a mile long whom he wanted me to meet.

The list included Chris McPeck, Michael Ramos and Dennis Craig, and these introductions continued until we headed to lunch with a family, the Flanigans, who touched my heart.

They arrived in my life and immediately entered my heart with their kindness, love, support and other amazing human qualities that I wanted to emulate.

There are just some people in your life who come in the front door, shut it behind them, and throw away the key. They were to be a part of my life forever more.

I remember staying with a family called the Hausos. Their son, Christopher, was the second baseman for the American team, and I was the second baseman for the Australian team.

Not only did we become friends, we became best mates to the point that he was in my wedding party nearly 10 years later. I quickly began to realise that this baseball program was far more than just a tour where young athletes get a chance to play baseball. This was a tour about life, about friendship, and about bringing people from other parts of the world together.

My return from my first trip to the US with the Expos marked an epoch in my life. I felt as though I had returned home as a young man; I was not a little boy anymore. I was of the conviction that anything was possible, and I began to feel very confident in my own skin and in my own ability. My friendships at school had begun to blossom, and I was at a point in my life where I was just so happy and content in the life that I was in.

I remember building up to the year 10 formal, which is a very big event on any high school student's social calendar. It was all about impressing, looking your best and having a great time. I remember asking one particular girl whether she would be my date for the formal. When she said yes, I was absolutely delighted.

The next day, she asked me whether her friend could join us. My immediate thought was: 'How good is it going to look to the boys when I show up with two girls?'

A few days later, I remember hearing that another girl didn't have a date for the formal, so I decided to ask the two girls whom I was taking whether she could join us for an hour.

The girls said they were happy for this to happen. So, my year 10 formal was going to be an absolute beauty. I had organised a nice hire suit, my aunt was going to drive us in a fancy car, and we were going to get plenty of photos when I showed up to the formal with my three ladies.

Two days prior to the formal, I got very unwell and was bedridden, but I was going to make sure that I had the energy to attend the formal. I remember getting out of bed late in the afternoon that day, putting on my suit, and driving to pick up the girls. We went to the headland and got some photos, and later, we arrived at the venue for a few more photos.

We walked up the stairs to greet a few people, but I then took the exit straight outside to get into the car to head home, as my body would not let me keep going. I desperately needed more rest.

It would have been an amazing night with the rest of my classmates, but at least I managed to show up, make an entrance and get some photos — and I got a few brownie points from the boys, because I showed up with three girls.

* * *

While I was in year 10 I was lucky enough to do work experience as a bellman at the Ritz-Carlton hotel in Sydney with my lifelong friend Wayne. (He was best mates with Nurse Jo's husband and we became great mates despite our 25 year age difference.) He had worked there for many years and was able to open up some doors (pardon the pun) and give me this opportunity. I remember taking people's bags to their rooms, opening doors and receiving tips from rich businessmen. One day I remember Greg Norman was staying and he gave me $20 to go to his penthouse and grab him four VBs, as the restaurant didn't serve that type of beer. Those two weeks of work experiences really shifted my mindset, and I thought to myself, 'One day I won't to be the guy that opens the door and receives the tips — I want to be the guy that has my door opened for me and for me to be in a position to give the tips.'

I was very pleased to make the Expos baseball team for the next two consecutive years, and it truly was a dream come true each year to be a part of this program. This game wasn't just a sport to me; it wasn't just something that we did on the weekend. It really became my life. These people in this Expo community were going to continue to help me live that dream.

* * *

I was 17 and had just finished my senior year at high school, and was still passionate about living the dream of playing baseball in America. Money had always been tight in our family, and if I wanted to play overseas I needed to pay my own way. My uncle Wayne Hosier ran an indoor air purification company selling the best vacuums on the planet. He offered me a role doing door-to-door sales, selling these $5500 vacuums. It was a commission-only role, so the harder I worked the more money I made. He made a deal with me when I started that if I could sell three machines in a week he would give me his beautiful Statesman to drive around for the weekend. I worked very hard, not only to sell and save but to also get the opportunity to drive that car. Let's just say my uncle didn't have his car very often on weekends! My time in Sydney living with my uncle and auntie and working with them was fast paced and extremely long hours, but I thoroughly enjoyed the challenge and, boy, did I make some money.

Just before my 18th birthday I was selected once again to play with the Expos in the United States. I was fortunate to play baseball down in Texas. A scout by the name of John Lee said to me in his thick, Southern accent: 'Son, you ain't the biggest ball player I have ever seen, but that passion you have certainly shines through. I want to give you an opportunity to come to Texas and play some college ball.'

I didn't know whether to cry or scream. I couldn't wait to get to a phone and call Mum to tell her what I thought was great news.

The phone call that I made that night was probably one of the toughest calls for me to make at this time in my life. She was pumped to hear my voice, but she was not so pumped to hear what I had to say.

I said to her: 'Guess what, Mum? I'm not coming home. I've been offered a scholarship to live here in Texas to play baseball for a college and also get an education.'

Mum's heart was so torn; she wanted her boy to come home, but she also wanted me to live my dream. Parents who truly love their children will move mountains and sacrifice their own yearnings and wishes in order to see their children live their dreams.

It's funny, because you move from Australia, where you're this little red-headed, skinny, freckly guy, and you've got a pretty awesome scar from where the cancer was cut out. None of the girls really wanted to talk to you back in Australia, and then, all of a sudden, you go to America and you speak with a funny accent, and suddenly you become really good-looking! My new-found confidence and my accent no doubt blurred their vision somewhat.

I didn't tell anybody in Texas that I'd been sick. You can imagine the stories that I made up about that scar because, in Texas, when you talk, people invariably say to you: 'Boy, you've got a funny accent. Where are you from?' I'd reply, 'I'm from Australia, mate.' You say it as fast as you can so no-one has a clue what you said.

They'd say, 'Australia? Nope, I've never heard of Australia. What state is Australia in?' You can tell them anything and they would believe you. I told them that my scar was from a mistimed jump off a paddleboat with Uncle Steve Irwin, which landed me on a crocodile's tail that cut me open. We would laugh and tell some wonderful stories.

They would believe me when I told them that I rode a kangaroo to school. My life was amazing; each morning I was so excited to simply get out of bed. I would sometimes pinch myself and think: 'Is this really happening to me?' I was making great friends, I was playing great baseball, and I was feeling so blessed to have the life that I had.

I had never wanted people to know about my health, because I never wanted to be treated any differently from the others. But, like everything in life, you can reach a pinnacle, and it can all get taken away from you in a heartbeat. I was 18 years old and I was certainly living the dream. But one bad choice, one bad decision, or even a phone call, and your life can change forever.

One day, I was playing a game in Arizona on a very hot Thursday night; the temperature was around 44 degrees Celsius at 8 pm. I slid into second base and I woke up three days later in hospital. My health was deteriorating, my immune system was getting weaker, and I suffered even more heart challenges.

My dreams that I had worked so hard for came to an end. My dreams of playing baseball in America were over.

Three weeks after getting out of the hospital, I was on the plane heading home. It took me 44 hours to get back to Coffs Harbour, and, I promise you, I cried 40 of those 44 hours, thinking that my life wasn't fair.

I thought: 'How many times do I need to get knocked and kicked?' I felt depressed, but there was this little feeling inside my heart of knowing that everything happens for a reason, and I was so excited to see my mum.

I'd had no idea how much I would miss her, and I had forgotten the enormous comfort she brings to me when time gets tough.

When I landed in Coffs Harbour, I remember getting off the plane, and thinking to myself that I had two choices. I could get off the plane and let everybody know that my dreams had been crushed: everyone would have understood it. They would have appreciated it. I could have got the sympathy vote for as long as I wanted it — or I could get off that plane with my head held high, knowing that I'd been able to achieve something far greater than what so many people thought I'd ever be able to achieve.

I got off the plane with the biggest smile on my face, and my tiny chest was puffed out, because I was proud of what I'd been able to do. There were two TV reporters there to greet me. The first reporter was from *A Current Affair*.

The reporter said: 'Mike, we want to do a story about your life. We think it's unfair what happened to you. We're going to do a three-minute story about your life.' Then she said that they would pay me $30 000 to do it.

I didn't care whether it was 30 seconds. I was an 18-year-old boy, with a large medical bill in the United States to pay, and I had no job and no car. In the split second after I heard the figure, I'd already picked out the car I was going to buy with my $30 000.

Fast and the furious was the fashion in cars back in those days. It was going to be a VN Holden Commodore Club Sport. It was going to be lowered, have 18-inch rims, have neon lights underneath, and the boot was going to have the biggest speaker that you've ever seen.

I wouldn't be able to fit my putter in there, let alone my golf bag. I was going to drive down the main street in the middle of winter, heater on, windows down, music pumping. I was going to be the biggest bogan in Coffs Harbour. Life was going to be awesome.

Then another TV producer approached me, snapping me out of my daydream. They said: 'Michael, we want to do a 30-minute story about your life. We're from *Australian Story*. We want to give you an opportunity to give back and make a difference.'

A Current Affair were offering $30 000 for three minutes. So, I am sure you can imagine what I was thinking: I just carried the zero to make it 30 minutes, and came to the logical amount of $300 000. How good was this going to be? I've gone from a VN Commodore to a Mercedes-Benz. I've gone from 18-inch to 20-inch rims!

I wasn't going to be just a bogan anymore; I was going to be a rich bogan. I was going to look after my mum. Life was going to be amazing.

I said: 'How much?', just wanting to confirm the maths.

They replied, 'Here at *Australian Story*, we don't pay for our programs. We do something far greater than that.'

That's when the 18-year-old brain pretty much switched off. I didn't care what they had to say; all I was thinking of was the car.

At that time, I was heavily involved with Camp Quality. There was a man from all those years ago who was literally standing by my side at the airport, having arrived with over

100 others to welcome me home: my dear friend (and former head of Camp Quality in my area), Tom Strickland. He said to me: 'Michael, here's your opportunity to give back. Here's your opportunity to make a difference in other people's lives as opposed to just trying to gain for yourself.'

So, that's what I did. I'm so blessed and so privileged to have been a part of *Australian Story*, in an episode called 'Field of Dreams'.

I remember day one of the filming. The camera crew arrived at my family home. They were all so kind and so caring and a bond was immediately formed. I remember the producer so clearly; her name was Janine Hoskins, and she said that she and her colleagues were so excited to be able to share my wonderful story.

We remain friends to this day, and I think that it was not so much my story but the way she produced it and shared it that made it such a great success. They followed me around for weeks and filmed some of my day-to-day routine, which included training and other activities, such as visits to the doctor and hospital.

I remember listening in my room one day as they interviewed my mum. They asked her to recall my time as a child and the challenges that she'd faced. I remember sitting there listening intently as tears flowed down my face; it broke my heart listening to the pain and the suffering that she went through watching me have my treatment, and hearing how she felt so helpless and just wanted to take my pain away every day, but simply couldn't do anything to help.

She shared some of her stories that she would write in her diary every day. I walked in her shoes just for an hour throughout that interview and I learned so much — not only about myself and my story, but also about the courage, the determination and her absolute refusal to ever quit on her little boy.

Somehow, that day my love, respect and admiration for my mother peaked at an all-time high, and I was so grateful for everything she had done and the sacrifices that she had made.

To be told, over and over again, to just walk away and quit, but to still keep fighting, was so admirable. I can only think how difficult she would have been considered by all the nurses, since she never took no for an answer. I am so glad she didn't.

It was even amazing listening to my three sisters share how it was for them and the challenges they went through with not only having their brother away for so long, but, more importantly, not having their mum there with them as they grew from little girls into young teenagers.

It was an emotional roller-coaster, but it had certainly become an exciting one, because we were finally all home together, and we shared some wonderful memories and crazy stories.

IF WE CHASE
POWER, PRIVILEGES
AND POSSESSIONS

$ WE MAY END UP
FINANCIALLY
RICH

YET EMOTIONALLY
POOR.

9

SO BEGAN MY CAREER – OR WAS IT

After the *Australian Story* aired on national TV, life became exciting for me. Lots of people started to recognise me when I walked down the street; many of them approached me, and asked to get their photo taken with me. I was asked to attend different events and share a little of my journey. I remember one company flew me in a private plane to their conference on the Gold Coast to sit and do a Q&A with their attendees.

But it did not last forever: the hype gradually faded, and at that stage, I was really a little lost. I had no job, no career, and no real direction. I managed somehow to start dating a young girl who was a cheerleader/dancer, Renee, so I thought I was 'the man'. I then moved to Newcastle and I got a job in finance, which was an industry I thought was awesome at the time. That career consumed me for many years.

At first, I got a job as the guy who stands at the front of the bank and welcomes you when you walk in. I had no idea about anything. My answer to every single question to every single customer was: 'Yeah; no problem. Just make your way over to the teller and they'll be able to help you out.' Whether the customer wanted a term deposit, a new account, or something else, my response was always: 'Make your way over to the tellers and they will be able to help you out.'

I gradually worked my way up into a position as a lender, and I began to learn very quickly that the more effectively you communicate, and the stronger the relationships you build, the greater the amount of products you can sell.

I truly believed in what I was offering; I felt that I was helping people to get closer to their dreams, get out of jams, and I was even putting them in a better financial position. It's amazing what happens when you really believe in a product; it really does sell itself.

I was building a great name for myself in the finance sector. I was the leader of all internal competition, I was making good money, and I had made some really great relationships that became life long friendships. Baseball competition was solid in the Newcastle area. I had a great team that was very competitive, and life was rolling along smoothly.

One day a man came into my work and greeted me. He said his name was Tom, and he even addressed me by my name. I was pretty impressed that he knew my name, but then I realised that I was wearing a name badge. I replied: 'Yes?'

He said, 'I'm the CEO; let's have a chat.'

I went into the back room to get him a coffee, and on my way out there, I asked a female colleague who Tom was. She informed me that he was the CEO. I had no idea what a CEO was, so I asked her to explain what he did.

She informed me that CEO stands for Chief Executive Officer, which just made me even more confused, so I asked what that title meant, and she explained that he was the boss's boss's boss's boss. I thought to myself: 'This guy must be rich, and I really need to impress him.' So, I sat down, feeling a bit nervous all of a sudden, because Tom was the big boss.

He said to me, 'Michael, where do you see yourself in five years?'

I was 19. All I cared about at that stage was where I was on a Friday night. I didn't care where I was going to be in five years. I didn't even know where I was going to be tomorrow.

I said to myself, 'Could I be cheeky here and get away with it? Let's have a crack.' So, I replied: 'Tom, I'm going to work hard over the next five years, and I am going to take your job.'

He looked at me thoughtfully: 'Michael, I don't know whether you're arrogant or determined, but only time will tell.'

That's when my 19-year-old self should have shut up, but my response to that was: 'Yes; you're right, Tom. Only time will tell.'

We didn't really get off on the right foot, but we eventually became good mates.

Within 12 months, I was a 20-year-old branch manager. This had its challenges, because my girlfriend and I were living in Newcastle and this role was a two-and-a-half-hour drive north to Port Macquarie.

I left home at 5.30 am every day, and arrived close to 8 am. I would work all day trying to impress my staff, who were not only much more experienced than I was, but possessed a far greater knowledge of both the industry and the area.

I would then drive home each afternoon, settling back into our home close to 8.30 pm. I understood the sacrifices that were required to get ahead in life.

My family never had money, could never afford to go on holidays or drive a nice car, and we would never have a fancy meal out and about. I really wanted these things for my future family: I wanted to be the provider, and I wanted nice cars and a nice house. But in retrospect, I think that I really just wanted the image that people paint of success.

With all of the travel and the pressure of getting the branch in a very lucrative position, I needed to commit more time to my work, which meant not driving home each day.

So, I started driving up on Mondays, travelling home on Wednesday nights, driving back up on Thursdays, and then driving home on Fridays for the weekend. While away from home I stayed with my amazing friends Michael and Cassie Pelley. This routine worked better, but it was still starting to strain the body and the mind.

Throughout this period of my life, I was still experiencing plenty of personal challenges, and my sister was separating from her husband. Then something happened that completely shattered my heart, and still shatters my heart to this day. My parents separated; they became one of the 80-plus per cent of separated parents of children with cancer.

My mum was heartbroken; she was so lost, and she was really struggling to find her purpose. It's truly awful when you see someone you care about in so much pain, and there is nothing that you really can do to support her or take her pain away.

It made me reflect on the pain she must have felt watching me battle for so long.

With all that was going on at home with my family and the struggles at work, the stress to my already beaten body was just too much to handle, and I was rushed to hospital with an illness that they could not identify.

After seven lumbar punctures over seven days, they transferred me from Maitland Hospital to the John Hunter Hospital. I was put in the palliative care unit, as this was the only ward that had a free room that was isolated. You can imagine the fear on beautiful Nurse Jo's face when she called to check in on me only to find that I was in the palliative care unit.

She hung the phone up and immediately drove from Sydney straight to Newcastle. Jo arrived and simply did what Jo does best. She made things happen. Finally, 24 hours after Nurse Jo arrived, I was diagnosed with bacterial meningitis.

I had a large amount of fluid on the brain, and I had never felt so sick, with so little energy and so much pain. It was a long stint in hospital, and yet again, the frustration of being stuck in the same bed, eating the same food, and having no choice about how to organise my days started to build up.

I was very fortunate to have some great friends who would visit me in hospital every day. Brad Garland, my baseball mate, would bring me food, magazines and plenty of laughs to lift my spirit.

My coach at the time, Nick, and his lovely wife would visit every second day. He owned several fruit shops, and each time they would bring a punnet of strawberries; they would have this big smile on their faces when they said, 'We brought you strawberries.' I didn't have the heart to tell them that I didn't like strawberries — but the nurses and doctors loved them.

I finally got out of hospital, and I tried to hit the ground running. Very quickly, I began to realise that the life I was living, the hours at work, and the challenges with my family, were taking a huge toll on my relationship with Renee, and after many years together, we went our separate ways. I recall many nights of tears, feeling so alone, and I questioned why all of these things were happening to me all at once.

But I truly believe that we are tested every day, and with great adversity comes not only great strength, but also new ideas and opportunities.

Several months after getting back on my feet, I was promoted to the largest and most under-performing site in the country. I was moving to Parramatta, in the big smoke, and this was an opportunity to put the past behind me and to work hard to get to the top of the corporate ladder. But I did not go there alone; my angel came with me.

Let me take you back to when I had just returned home from the States from a baseball tour when I was 17. My angel entered my world at a young age, even though at the time, I had no idea of the impact she would have on my life.

She was at an auction with her father and I don't know why I was there, but as I wandered through all of the items that were up for auction, I saw a beautiful young girl walk past me. Her hair was flying in the wind.

Her smile instantly brought warmth and joy into my life. I remember she walked past and I said, 'Hello.' She said 'Hi' back and we started chatting. It felt so comfortable, so right, so real. At this time, I didn't know how old she was. I just thought that she was beautiful.

I remember going home that afternoon and saying to my sister, 'I met an angel today.'

She said to me, 'Did you get her number?' I said that I didn't know why I didn't get her number, but I didn't. About two weeks later, I received a phone call from an unknown number, and the voice said, 'Hi, it's Mel. I met you at the auction.'

I was so delighted and excited to hear her voice, because I couldn't track her number down, but she had tracked mine. I immediately arranged to catch up with her for lunch on a Sunday and we had an amazing afternoon of chatting and laughing before I drove her home. When I dropped her off she said to me, 'Would you like to pick me up from school tomorrow?' I said that I would love to.

In the back of my mind I was interested to know how old she was, purely because she was still at school. I was 17 and I thought she would be close to 17. I picked her up the next day from school and her uniform was a junior uniform, which as you can imagine, surprised me a lot, because I thought she was at least a senior.

Long story short, I found out that she was only in grade 9, and she was 14. We stayed friends for a very long time. In fact, for six or seven years we stayed friends until our lives eventually came together once more, and not only were we friends, but we became soulmates. Our lives connected again. She made the first move with me and we've been inseparable ever since.

So we embarked on this exciting journey together: she knows all of my stories, my challenges, and she is willing to make the best of the life we have. We made some amazing friends throughout our time in Sydney. We, like all couples, had our ups and downs, but she always supported me with everything that I embarked on.

Times were really challenging in the business world; the branch was underperforming, we had the wrong people working for the organisation, and I had to let a lot of people go. I think that the success of any business comes from its people, not its customers. The customers will come if you can create a great environment with products that you believe in.

I needed to have the right people in the right roles, and once we did, boy, did we fire to the top. Our numbers were out of control; we couldn't keep up with business, and the money was fantastic. I was living a life that I really had never thought would be possible: fancy cars, beautiful dinners, amazing holidays and the bank account was full. But it still wasn't enough.

I was promoted to a national role and travel became an everyday thing. I was losing friends, I was not enjoying the fake picture of success I had painted for everybody to see, and the worst of it all was that my relationship with Mel began to suffer. I became very depressed and would cry daily about the life that I had created.

I had painted the 'perfect' picture of success. We had the sports cars, the fancy apartment and the big bank account, but I had an empty heart. I was missing my partner, missing my family and some days I just didn't really want to get out of bed. I realised that I could keep pushing up the corporate ladder, making more money and buying nicer things, but I'd probably end up broken and alone.

I realised my priorities, and that was my family, so we both decided to move back to Coffs Harbour to be closer to them. I was offered the bank manager job for Westpac, and I thought that this could really assist us with stability and allow us to start fresh, close to our old friends.

Things started very well for both of us. Mel had a steady job and I was enjoying my wonderful new team in Coffs Harbour. One day, I decided to make the ultimate commitment by asking for Mel's hand in marriage.

It was the hardest conversation I had ever had at that point in my life when I asked her father, Steve, whether I could marry his beautiful daughter. Steve and I bumped heads a lot, unfortunately. I just wanted him to like me, but I think that we may have been too similar in terms of our desire to succeed in the corporate world, so we clashed a little, which made the question even harder, although we have since become great friends.

I finally built up the courage to ask him as I was racing to the airport, which was not the greatest of places to ask. If I had my time over, I would have really made more effort, because I truly loved his daughter more than anything in the world. Despite the rockiness of the conversation, I got his approval and we flew to Bali on a little getaway.

I had only picked up the ring on my way to the airport after locking it away in my mum's cupboard for safe keeping and so no snoopers (i.e. Mel) would find it. We arrived at the airport and I realised that I still had the ring box in the top pocket of my jeans, and thought that if I went through security with her and had to take it out, she would see it and the surprise would have been over. Panicking, I sent her in before me to start checking in and managed to open up the luggage and sneak it into a pair of socks.

I had hired a restaurant in the hills of Ubud, and there were candles and rose petals everywhere. As a cover artist started singing one of Mel's favourite Michael Bublé songs, I got down on one knee and asked her to make me the happiest man on the planet. 'You are my life; will you be my wife?'

She said yes.

We came home from our holiday and celebrated with all our family and friends. We had two amazing engagement parties: one in Coffs Harbour with our wonderful friends and family, and then another gathering in Sydney.

But then it was back to work. Westpac gave me an opportunity to stretch, and again, I was burning the candle at both ends. I had five sites to juggle, and the ongoing roles of keeping my staff, my family and Mel happy.

I felt as though I was failing in all departments. The dark thoughts of depression kicked back in, and I was not enjoying life. From the outside in, I looked as though I had it made. I had a beautiful soon-to-be wife, lovely home, great car, awesome job, and I was surrounded by great people. But inside, I was alone; I was lost and I was stressed.

I think that stress is something that is crippling and debilitating. It's something that can suck you down and hold on to you for as long as you let it. People say that positive thinking can help reduce stress and sometimes dissolve it altogether. My opinion is that positive thinking doesn't mean that you keep your head in the sand and ignore life's less pleasant situations. Positive thinking just means that you approach unpleasantness in a more positive and productive way.

You think the best is going to happen, not the worst. Positive thinking often starts with self-talk, which is the endless stream of unspoken thoughts that run through your head. These automatic thoughts can be positive or negative.

Some of your self-talk comes from logic and reason. Other self-talk may arise from misconceptions that you create because of lack of information. If the thoughts that run through your head are mostly negative, your outlook on life is more likely to be pessimistic.

If your thoughts are mostly positive, you're likely an optimist. But at this point in my life, I was only looking at the glass that was half empty, not the glass that was half full. I was Mr Pessimistic, and I had lost clarity, direction and purpose.

But why, after all that I had been through? I think it was that I had worked so hard to reach a certain level in the corporate field, which I thought was going to bring me joy and happiness, but it only brought me money and stress.

One afternoon when I was at the office, I started to feel horrible and my head started to pound; my neck was sore, my eyes were aching, and then I realised I was drooling out the side of my mouth.

My PA came in and said, 'What's happened to your face?' It had dropped down on the right side. I was taken to hospital and was informed that I had Bell's Palsy, which is almost like a stroke that affected me on my right side.

I was a little lost soul. I would not talk to anyone, I didn't want visitors, and when Mel would leave the room of a night time, I would pray.

It was not the same prayer that I'd said when I was a child who just wanted to go home and get out of the hospital; it was something much darker than that. It hurts me to think that I was ever in a place to pray for this, but I did. Each night, I would pray to God that I would not wake up in the morning. I didn't want to face the challenges anymore, I didn't want to be sick or stressed; I just wanted to rest and be at peace. But God never listened and I kept waking up each morning. Day by day, I got stronger and stronger, not only physically, but more importantly, mentally.

I REFLECT AND THINK
LIFE IS SO SHORT;

IF YOU'RE NOT LOVING WHO YOU ARE AND WHAT YOU'RE DOING,

THEN MAKE THE CHANGE TO BECOME YOUR BEST.

#1

(10)
LIVING INTO
MY LEGACY

When I got out of hospital, I made the bold decision to walk away from the corporate life and to follow my dream of making a global impact as an inspirational speaker, sharing my thoughts, ideas and stories with the world. People laughed, and others told me that I was crazy to walk away from a wonderful career to follow something that sounded so unsubstantial and flaky. Yet, I think in life that is part of the fun: simply not knowing what is around the corner.

I needed to master a few things in life: I needed to master the gift of giving. I needed to truly understand what success was, and I needed to begin to live into my legacy.

I had the support of my fiancée to walk away from a very healthy salary to follow a goal and a vision, where our futures were completely uncertain, and with no idea at all as to where it would lead us.

Still, I thought I needed to give back in areas where I thought I could make a difference. I was sitting in my lounge room when I realised the answer was staring me in the face: on the wall there was a picture of me with some friends at Camp Quality as a child. I thought: 'I am going to become a companion and spend time with these little angels who are coping with so much and dealing with something that I completely understand.'

Camp Quality gave me so much for so long, and now I was finally in a position to give back. I had plenty of time, and I took Mel along with me to Camp Quality and we both became companions.

On my first camp, a little boy came up to me and gave me a big hug. He had been very unwell. His name was Christian, and I remember the day that I met this little guy, I knew that he was going to be a part of my life forever. He brought such happiness into my life.

I reflect back on my own experiences as a child with my own Camp Quality companion, and I hope that this was the same happiness that I brought to my companion, Simon, back in the 1980s.

© Damien Ford Photography

Former CEO of Camp Quality Simon Rountree and I with the Camp Quality puppets as I'm announced as the new National Ambassador.

I was inspired by Christian's courage, optimism, and his smiles. I reflect on so many things throughout my life when somebody has given to me, and it's made me feel good, but when I have given to them or given to someone else, the feeling is so much greater. I think that the saying 'You receive far more from giving than you'll ever receive from receiving' is so true.

The happiness and the joy that it brings to you when making a difference to others is so much better than when somebody makes a difference to you. We had so many fun times on camp.

Christian was the camp prankster; he loved to prank anybody and everybody all the time. I remember on my first camp, he was going around putting little cups of flour on the tops of all of the doors, so that when people walked into the room, they would open the door and a cup of flour would fall on them.

He laced the top of the fan in my room one day with flour. When it got really hot, I turned the fan on and flour went everywhere in the room. Somehow, he managed to catch a wild turkey and put it in my room, and when I came into the room at night, there was a crazy turkey sitting on my bed.

He filled up my sleeping bag with Weet-Bix and corn flakes, and I remember one day he put cling wrap over the toilet, so when I raced to the toilet, I wasn't going into the toilet. To hear his laughter and to hear the joy in his voice — to see him be a normal kid and just have fun — demonstrates so powerfully and so beautifully the impact that Camp Quality has on so many different people.

Today, I'm still Christian's companion, but he's much more than that; he is my friend and always will be. He's healthy and he's happy and it's so wonderful to be a part of his journey.

In 2012, I became the National Ambassador for Camp Quality, which makes me a large part of so many different fundraising events around the country.

I'm very proud to say, my contribution has resulted in over $1 000 000 that has been raised for this great charity. I believe it costs $880 to send a child to Camp Quality each year, so I think about the $1 000 000-plus raised, and I realise that it is a lot of kids who are getting a great opportunity to be a part of something so special.

Camp Quality also helped me to break into the speaking world. I think to really make it in the speaking world you need a thick skin and a relentless determination to simply be able to break down the barriers and get on stage to share your message. But there's always that underlying importance of being at the right place at the right time.

One day, I received a phone call from the CEO of Camp Quality at the time, Simon Rountree. He said: 'Michael, we're wondering whether you would be available to share your journey with the Canterbury Bulldogs NRL team?' I was so excited and could not wait to seize this opportunity as I love Rugby League, even though I did not know much about the Bulldogs or their players.

I made sure that I was available and got on the plane to speak to the team. I called a friend of mine, Simon O'Dell, who came along to film the presentation, as this was a massive step into the professional sporting world for me.

We arrived at the auditorium and set up. I remember Des Hasler, the head coach, walked in and said: 'Michael are you ready to go, you all good, you need anything, you're ready, is it all good?' He was an intense character who spoke very fast, but he was extremely passionate about this game, so I was pumped and ready!

When everybody arrived, I realised that there were no players in attendance; it was only front office staff, management, board members and coaching staff. I've got to be honest and say that I was a little bit disappointed, but it was still a great opportunity to be a part of a very successful sporting team.

The presentation went very well. In fact, it went so well that Des and the CEO, Todd Greenberg, invited me back the following week to speak to all of the players. I remember sending a photo to my cousin, who has been a Bulldogs fan all his life, asking him whether he could tell me the names of the people who were in the photo with me; I had no idea who they were!

You can imagine that his response was rather explicit, because he would've done anything to be in that room with those players. The Bulldogs invited me to all of their home games, and I became very close friends with many of the players. I am not sure whether it was coincidence or luck, but from then on, they went on to achieve a 12-game winning streak and they made the grand final. I had to do the right thing by my cousin, Nathan, so I took him to the grand final game; otherwise he probably would have never forgiven me. Unfortunately, they were beaten, but what a wonderful experience to be a part of that journey.

I still continue to interact with this club and their players to this day. I now maintain such strong relationships and bonds with Trent Hodkinson, Josh Reynolds, Josh Morris, and Mick Ennis, who is a real blessing. And it all came off the back of this amazing organisation, Camp Quality. To be in and around the club during the transformation that it had in those days was phenomenal.

Still, as you know, my passion has always been baseball, and to be able to speak to baseball players and professional athletes would be a real dream come true.

I was speaking to all of the athletes at a college in the United States when a gentleman said to me: 'Michael, I'm going to arrange for you to speak to the Toronto Blue Jays.' If I had a dollar for every time someone had offered me to speak somewhere, life would be very different. Unfortunately, many people will offer you the world and deliver you absolutely nothing.

This has happened to me over and over again. I get that on a regular basis because I get caught up in the excitement of other people's ideas and connections, which sadly, often lead nowhere! So, I thanked him for his kind offer and thought to myself: 'Yup; just another offer that will go nowhere.' This guy's name was Steve Springer, and to be honest, I had no idea who he was.

But he was a man of his word, and he was going to make this happen. After doing a little research, I realised that he had played in the big leagues and he was now the hitting coach for some of the best hitters in Major League Baseball.

I can't tell you the sheer excitement that ran through my veins, nor the exhilaration and pride of my family, when I received an email from the Blue Jays asking for my availability during their spring training camp in March. I realised that mixing my love of baseball with my career as a speaker was really going to happen.

The flight was long and flying economy class was a little uncomfortable, yet those things were put aside and overtaken by the sheer excitement of getting a chance to spend time with some of the best baseball players on the planet. Arriving at Spring Training camp, seeing the freshly cut grass, the perfectly aligned field, and the amazing stadium, was indescribable.

I had goosebumps, and it was almost like something I had worked so hard for and for so long had finally come true. Meeting the coaching staff, front office employees and then the players: what an experience that was. And then, as if that was not enough, I had the opportunity to share my journey with them on stage.

I had the chance to throw at batting practice, and spend time on the field. I also got to go out for dinner with them, which was a real treat and a memory that I will treasure for a lifetime. It's awesome years later that I still have these people in my life, and I still have the opportunity to go back to Spring Training every year.

In 2015 I had a very special trip to Spring Training, because I spent time with one of my sporting idols whose turn double plays I used to watch when I was in hospital in Sydney; my mum always tried to tape the games that he played in.

His name was Roberto Alomar. The day he came to Spring Training, drove me around in his Bentley, and went out to lunch with me, was certainly a highlight of my life. The Blue Jays made it all the way through the play-offs and just missed out on playing in the World Series; what an amazing experience to have been a part of that ride!

One day, I was asked to speak at a conference in Denver, Colorado. I hoped it was going to open many doors and give me great exposure in the American market (I later realised that was not the case), and they said, 'We have no budget, but we really want these kids to hear your story.'

So I decided to make the journey to the other side of the world to share my story with these underprivileged college students. What I didn't realise was that this was going to change my outlook on life forever.

After a very long trip, I finally arrived in Denver, went to the hotel, checked in, had a quick shower, and went downstairs to share my story with the audience. It was the longest Q&A session post presentation that I have ever had. These kids were so engaged. I was so present; they were like sponges and just wanted to learn and soak up everything I had to give them.

Receiving a standing ovation in front of 15 000 people at the MGM Grand in Las Vegas, late 2019.

I found out while I was there that the total combined income for parents of the students attending this event could not be more than $20 000 a year. These were kids that are faced with some pretty nasty challenges, and it really became an honour to make an impact on these kids' lives.

After I left Denver, it was a long flight back to Australia, and three weeks went by during which I continually thought about these amazing people who were just so passionate about life. One day, I received a letter in the mail.

The letter began with the line: 'I use the rope to play tug-of-war.' It was a letter from a young lady who had been sitting in the front row in Denver, whom I recalled very clearly, thanks to her description of herself as 'the big Gothic girl in the front row'. She had been wearing lots of black make-up; her nail varnish was black, her dress was black, and she was the picture of what many people categorise as Goth.

In the letter she went on to tell me that she had been raped by her father, and when she told her mother she was bashed repeatedly, because the mother thought that she was lying and was trying to cause drama within the family.

She really didn't fit in at her college, she didn't have many friends, and she really just didn't connect well with the world. The morning of my presentation, she'd gone to the local hardware store and bought a long piece of rope and tied it up in her room inside the cupboard.

There was a knock on her door, and it was one of the teachers informing her that she must come down to hear a guy from Australia speak, but she told the teacher that she was not feeling well and that she was going to stay in her room.

She was going to do the unthinkable. The teacher persisted and insisted that she go downstairs to hear the Australian man speak, because he had flown a long way to be there, so everyone needed to attend. So as frustrated and angry as she was, she went downstairs to listen to my speech.

In her letter to me, she said that something changed in her mind about ending her life prematurely; she had gotten greater clarity around her purpose, and she went on to tell me that she realised her adversity, her pain and her challenges in life did not need to define her, but could instead give her strength to appreciate the finer things in life.

So, rather than going back to her room to kill herself after my talk, she decided to untie the rope, and head downstairs to play tug-of-war with all the other kids. Because she was a large girl, everybody wanted her on their team; she became the anchor and they won every challenge. Hence the opening line in her email to me, 'I use the rope to play tug-of-war'.

She said that day had changed her life. The other kids realised that she was a lovely girl, and just because she dressed differently, it didn't make her a bad person.

I reflect on this letter regularly and I think to myself how lucky I am to be in the position I am: by simply sharing my adversities, my challenges and my stories, I can have a positive impact on others, and I may even save someone's life.

I want people to understand that it's not materialistic possessions and money that change people; it can be something as simple as a smile. Smiling is one of the special abilities that is associated with being human.

It is the best way to express a great mood, and it is a powerful way to share these happy feelings with others. Smiling also functions as a symbol to express love, friendship, and care; it is recognised by others as something that comes from your heart. Some people say that smiling is contagious, because no-one wants to live in an unhappy world; they prefer to spend their time around those people who always wear a smile on their face and with people who can enjoy a great laugh.

There is a saying that smiling makes you live longer, because it will lead us to healthier and happier living. We can attain more health benefits in smiling, too. Most of the doctors who treated me said that laughter is the best medicine, just like Camp Quality's motto.

For me, a smile also reduces stress and makes me much more relaxed. Giving the sweetest smile to someone will ease his or her problems and loneliness and will cost you absolutely nothing. I think that it also strengthens our immune system, which is certainly something very important for me.

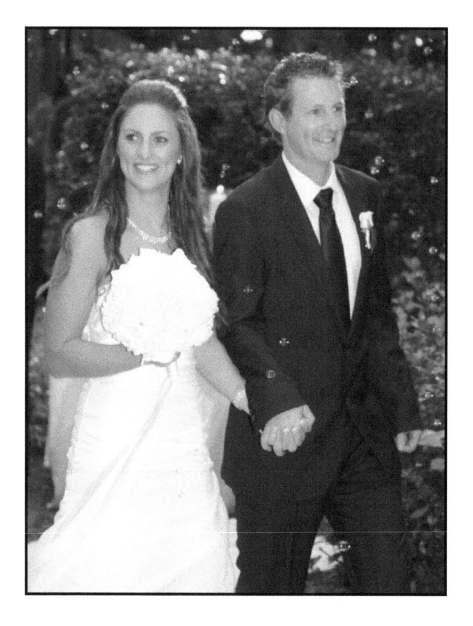

Mel and I on our wedding day, 21 April 2012.

A smile is the ambassador of your goodwill. It brightens up the lives of those people who see someone smiling at them. It is like a sunrise that gives light to the darkest of days. I often like to pose the following question to people:'What am I? I cost nothing, but I create much. I enrich those who receive me, without impoverishing those who give me. I happen in a flash, but their memory of me sometimes lasts a lifetime.' Your smile can be a game changer.

* * *

In April 2012, after several trips to the States speaking, Mel and I finally had enough money to get married. It was such a special day at the beautiful Bonville Golf Resort among wonderful family and friends. Later that year, we went on our honeymoon to Fiji for seven nights.

Unfortunately, I spent six of the seven nights in bed sick. I became very unwell after a big speaking tour and my body was exhausted. Still, I was not alone; I had my beautiful wife playing nurse and looking after me.

She would sunbake on the balcony, and I would rest up in the shade. It really hit me throughout our honeymoon just how lucky I am to have this amazing wife a part of my life forever.

We then travelled to the States for two weeks to spend time with friends who now feel like family. It was a really wonderful trip, and it allowed us to truly be together and to be truly present with each other.

MASTER
THE GIFT
OF GIVING

AND
YOU
WILL

MASTER
THE GIFT
OF LIFE.

*

11
THE POWER
OF GIVING

When we returned home from our honeymoon, we bought ourselves a nice home in sunny Sawtell. We loved the location, because it is close to beaches, and our family and friends. The house was no mansion; it was a modest four-bedroom home and was all that we required. It was on a nice large block and we loved the backyard.

One day, Mel asked me whether we could get a fireplace. I've always been taught that a good husband says two words that we must understand clearly, and those two words are: 'Yes, dear.' So needless to say, we got the fireplace. But I am not handy. In fact, I'm probably on the other end of the spectrum of 'handy'; I am hopeless when it comes to either building or fixing things.

We hired a friend to come around to install the fireplace. He eventually got to the point where he was putting in the down pipe, and he asked me whether I could give him a hand. I, of course, jumped to his aid, and said, 'What can I do?'

He asked me whether I could just catch the stainless steel pipe and put it into place as he lowered it from the roof. Unfortunately, when he was reaching down from the roof, he dropped it and it severed the tendons, nerves and ligaments in my thumb! Blood went everywhere and made an absolute mess. He drove me straight to the hospital and, fortunately enough, I'm pretty well known there, because I've spent a lot of time there. I went straight into surgery.

While waiting to go in, I noticed a little boy with a big smile on his face lying next to me in another bed. I thought that this was quite strange as everybody in this room was going into surgery. I guess the morphine had really kicked in. A nurse walked in and pulled the sheets back to see what his issue was, and she said: 'Oh, my God! What has happened to you?'

The little boy went on to tell the nurse what had happened. He said that he had been riding his quad bike through the bush, he had fallen off it, and a stick had lodged itself into his leg. Yet, he finished the sentence with something that I thought was pretty powerful. He finished by saying, 'But nurse, it could be worse.'

The nurse immediately questioned his logic and queried how it could possibly be worse: 'You have a stick in your leg, you aren't going to be able to go swimming, you will be on crutches, you will have to have surgery; what do you mean it could be worse?'

Still, the little boy with the big smile on his face insisted to the nurse that it could have been worse: 'The stick could have got me in the balls.' I roared laughing and so did everybody else in the room, including the nurse. I can just imagine the father saying to the little boy on the way to the hospital: 'Son, quit your whingeing; the stick could've got you in the balls!', and immediately, he would have stopped crying.

Not only is this a very funny story, but I feel that this story is so much deeper than is initially apparent. I think that what this little boy said is something so true, and his message is something for us all to live our lives by. Regardless of our adversities, our pain, and our suffering, it could always be worse, and it's not our adversity that defines us, but rather, it's all about how we deal with it.

All we need to do these days is to switch on the TV to see how much hatred and pain is in the world. From people killing others at pubs, kids bullying other kids and divorce rates skyrocketing, to the horrible and heartbreaking terrorist attacks that are destroying entire communities and countries forever, it is so clear that our own adversities could be far worse. We need to appreciate each day and learn to not only love one another, but to also give back to the world.

Over the course of my journey I started to realise that I could not settle for just travelling, speaking, sharing, and using the power of a smile with anybody and everybody; I needed something more. I needed to master the power and the gift of giving. I needed others to realise that, regardless of whether you're the rich guy or the poor guy, we all have the same opportunity to give, whether it's helping an old lady across the road, helping someone to unpack their trolley full of groceries, or giving someone a smile. Something as simple as sharing a smile with somebody can really change someone's life. For me, that is how I really need to live my life.

Through the challenges that I continue to face, mastering the gift of giving was going to shape my future. Because for me, when I worked in the corporate world, I was very driven by the three Ps — the Power, the Privileges, and the Possessions — and even though I gained all of those, I wasn't happy. I wasn't enjoying life. And the one thing that I didn't focus on was happiness. When you start to shape your outlook on life purely around happiness, it's amazing what you can achieve.

I guess in life your dreams are one thing, but the reason behind those dreams is something far greater. The joy of accomplishing something is amazing. When you realise that you can help other people achieve similar dreams, it far outweighs the joy that you received when you achieved your own.

I continued to participate in the Aussie Expos Baseball program that had taken me to the States many times over in the past, and I became a member of the coaching staff.

Unfortunately, my dear friend, mentor and former coach, John Murray, passed away after years of sickness. The program was no longer going to continue.

That same year that the program was meant to cease, I made a promise to a little boy by the name of Sean Richards; he was a perfect stranger, but he was to later become a very important part of my family. He, unfortunately, had a very bad go-kart accident just before Christmas and was given two bits of news. The good news was he didn't have a broken back.

The bad news was they had found a tumour in his spine, and it didn't look good. I made a commitment to him to stay strong and to keep close to his side throughout his cancer battle. I promised him that I would take him to America, because like me, it was his dream to one day play baseball in America.

Obviously, the program couldn't finish when I'd made that commitment. I asked the Murray family whether they would allow me to continue the program in honour of the legacy that their father had left. They agreed, and I was fortunate to be able to take this little boy to the United States to live his dreams. Just like me when I played over there as a child, he was definitely not the biggest or the fastest. He was, in fact, the smallest and probably the slowest, but we wanted to make sure his dream came true.

I remember putting him out onto the field. It was the last inning of the game. We were winning by two runs. We put him at second base, and all of a sudden, the American team started to swing the bat. Base hit here. Base hit there. Stolen base here. Extra base hit there. It was a 3–2 ballgame, with one out and loaded bases.

A young American boy stepped up to the plate and hit the ball hard into the gap between shortstop and third. The shortstop backhanded the ball and fired it over to Sean, who just happened to be standing on second base. We were hoping that the ball wouldn't hit him, but it managed to hit him all right: right in the middle of the glove. He caught the ball, and then to our immense joy and excitement, he stepped on second base.

We immediately thought: 'That's fabulous. Now they've scored a run and it's a three-all ball game, but there's two out. Hopefully, we can get the last out and go in the extra innings.' However, *Sean* had a different outcome in his mind. He stepped off second base.

He fired the ball to first, and he turned the game ending into a winning double play. Talk about tears of joy and tears of happiness! That was a moment in my life that I will never forget; it was a moment where I realised that I had just helped somebody else's dream come true, and it would change their life forever.

Now, I've been a part of that program and continue to be as the tour manager and director. I hope to continue the legacy that John Murray has left by helping others to live out their dream of playing baseball in America.

Two years ago, I was fortunate to take a boy by the name of Todd Nester. He was a contestant on the award-winning Australian TV show *The Biggest Loser*. He had lost 38 kilos in less than four months. I found out via that program that his dream was also to play baseball in America. It was a real treat to be able to take him over there and allow him to be a part of that program.

In summary of my baseball journey, it started off as a dream for me about what I could do as an athlete, and what I could do as a baseball player. Now, it's turned into something far greater than that. It's become a job where I can help, educate, hone skills, teach other people, and give other people the opportunity to live their dreams. For me, that is just a great joy and a great gift, which I'm lucky to share with so many people around the world now.

But that's not where the beginning stopped; instead, it was where the beginning started.

On 12 January 2010, an earthquake hit Haiti. It killed approximately 316 000 people, and it left millions of people homeless. Haiti is around one third of the size of Tasmania. Yet, it has a population of over 10 million people.

The devastation was absolutely abhorrent, and it made worldwide news. A significant amount of money was donated to Haiti to try to rescue them from the devastation. Unfortunately, a massive amount of corruption saw a lot of that money disappear. The support and the aid just never arrived.

In 2012, I was fortunate to venture down to Haiti with Cheryl and John Ward, who have become lifelong friends. When you experience something as graphic and heartbreaking as being in that environment, it changes you forever. Your outlook, your perspective, your thoughts on humankind definitely change.

You begin to ask a lot of questions: 'Why?', 'Why is the world the way that it is?', 'Why does devastation have to debilitate not only families, but communities, towns and an entire nation?'

I reflect back on my first time visiting Haiti. I flew from Coffs Harbour, the beautiful coastal town of northern New South Wales, and I landed in the busy city of Sydney. I flew from Sydney to Los Angeles, where there are millions and millions of people, and where there is wealth. I flew from Los Angeles to Miami, where wealth goes to an extreme level.

There are houses that are valued in the vicinity of US$15 to 20 million, which are sitting on the edge of pristine waterways. Then, I boarded a plane with 165 other people — 165 of whom were Haitians. I was the only white guy who got on the plane.

I landed in Port-au-Prince to be greeted by the smell of death, decaying bodies, sewage, the heat, the humidity, and the noise of people yelling and screaming as they saw me arrive, trying to grab me through the fence. I went through customs, and the man stared at me. He didn't say a word, but slammed the stamp down on my passport, and looked up, as if to say: 'Off you go.'

I arrived inside a little tin shed, where they throw your bags from the carousel onto the ground in a massive mound. People just dived in and grabbed their bags. I got my bag, and there were people with red shirts everywhere, trying to carry my bag out, so I gave them money. I just carried my own bag and I started walking out, knowing that there would be a man in a car, waiting for me to go.

I walked down a very narrow corridor, with a tin roof cover over the top, which was now outside. There was a barbed wire fence either side of me. I heard people yelling in Creole; they were spitting and trying to grab me as I walked right down the middle, so I felt a little safe.

I waited for 15 minutes; the traffic was horrendous, so my lift was late. When it arrived, I saw that the broken windows were replaced with plastic bags. As I got in, the smell of burning rubber and burning plastic just filled the air. We drove for miles and miles, and the depth of the devastation started to kick in.

My emotions took over, and I could not help but cry. I saw people who were completely and utterly helpless. They had nothing: no families, no roof over their heads. No drinking water. No place to even go to the bathroom. I saw young women, young boys and girls, urinating in the street, because there was nowhere else to go.

I could see people begging on the side of the street, their hands and their feet missing, with just bandages around them. Every time we would stop at traffic lights, there would be people knocking on the window, begging for money. The smell was something that I can't possibly explain in words. Your breath shortens, so as to minimise the horrific smell that consumes your nasal passages, your throat, and into your lungs. The traffic was worse than what you would see in central Los Angeles.

We were literally stationary for 15, 20, 25 and 30 minutes at a time, without the wheels rolling an inch. Every now and then, the car would get stuck where there was someone burning their rubbish. The smell of burnt plastic just wafted through, and I needed to wrap my face up with a jumper to try to take away the smell, so I could hardly breathe.

We arrived at a little shop, where we were going to get some food before we trekked up the mountain. We'd found out that many of the children who lived on the mountain were walking four or five hours a day, simply to try to get to school. Some of the things that were happening to them, not only on their way to school, but on their way home, were just horrific.

We felt that this was the place where we could add value. This was a place where we could go along to rebuild something very important, like a school, sparing the kids this epic daily trek. We'd try to break the mould, or break the cycle, and allow these people to get on their feet, so they could start to realise that they had a future. There is always hope, and there are people who genuinely care.

You reflect on days when you complained about how bad the traffic was, how uncomfortable your bed is sometimes, how hot you are, how cold you are, how you don't want to do an assignment, how you don't want to dial into that conference call, and how you don't really want to go to work today. You quickly realise, with a grinding shock, that your First World problems pale into insignificance compared with what these people face and experience every single day.

We drove for two hours to get to the base of where we started to trek. We went past crushed buildings, where there were just little crosses out the front of where the buildings had been. We found out that many of the bodies were still inside, because they didn't have the infrastructure to get them out. We began to trek up the mountain.

I finally met up with my Australian friends. The trek takes about 10 hours, and I knew that it was going to be a great challenge, because it was a very steep walk. We had to carry a lot of tools for the build. We got about an hour into the trek, and I said to one of the guys who was directing us: 'How far to go?' He replied: 'We're halfway.' I thought: 'Fantastic, we've only got an hour to go.'

Then what felt like another three hours went by, and I asked him, 'How far are we?' He said, 'Halfway.' We were four hours into the journey, and we were only halfway?

Our water supply was about a third gone. We got about six hours into the trek, and I asked the man, 'How far are we away?' He responded: 'We're halfway.' Now, I started to panic, because we had been trekking for six hours. He had told me that we were halfway, so my immediate thought was that we still had another six hours to go. I looked down, and my bottle of water was empty.

The temperature was around 42 degrees Celsius. I was very dehydrated. My knees started to ache. My ankles were sore. My heart was beating out of my chest, and all I could think of was having a cold drink.

We got to the base of the last climb, and there was a freshwater stream. Unfortunately, it was not fresh enough to drink, but it was certainly fresh enough to swim in. It reduced my body temperature and made me feel so much better. All the pain seemed to go away as my body temperature reduced.

When I got out of the water, they gave me a tin of tomato juice, because that was the only liquid that we had left. I cracked open the tin, had half a mouthful, and then I begin to vomit violently and profusely.

It was something that my body definitely did not need. I realised that all I needed to do was get to the site where we were building the school, so I would be able to get some fresh water. We were another hour in, so the trek had now gone for seven, nearly eight hours.

I asked my buddy, 'How far are we in?' He answered: 'We're halfway.' I realised, then and there, that's about all he could say in English: 'We're halfway.'

Finally, we stopped at a tiny little campsite, and there was a lady who had a familiar face. I was absolutely delighted, because she was there with a bottle of clean water. I wanted to drink it all, but I realised that there were many of us, and we were all very dehydrated. We passed the water around, and she assured us we only had one hour of climbing to go.

We were about 20 minutes into that last hour, and my body just seemed to begin to fail. There were seven little girls climbing with us, all carrying very heavy bottles of water on their heads. It was almost like there were seven little angels who just wouldn't leave me. I sat under a tree, because I needed to get some energy back, and so did they. I didn't want to get up, but they helped me up.

When the trek became narrow, they would stand behind me to help me up the hills. These beautiful little kids had just walked four hours down and four hours back to get some fresh water out of the pond, so that they had water they could drink (after taking it home and boiling it to try to kill all the germs). They walked beside me. They walked behind me. They walked with me all the way, until we got to the site where we were going to build the school. Then, they continued on to their village.

We got to a flat area, where the concrete had already been laid, and the view was breath-taking. Over the next two weeks, we battled the heat, the humidity, the lack of water every day, all day and all night. During the day, the temperatures got up to as high as 44 degrees Celsius, and of a night, it would get as low as 5 or 6 degrees.

It was a fascinating climate, because we would need to get changed into our bed clothes by 6 pm. Otherwise, it would get so cold that you would feel like you were going to catch pneumonia, even though, just a couple hours earlier, you were so hot you would just constantly sweat.

Two weeks went by, and we managed to build something that was so special. These kids no longer had to walk hours and hours of a day and a night to get an education; the school had come to them. The saying 'If you build it, they will come' was so true. Within the first week of opening, there were 120 kids attending the school. Within one year, we had 230 children going to this school every single day.

We have five full-time teachers, and a principal who lives onsite to support the kids. To see the impact of giving to other people is one of the greatest feelings of all.

I went to Haiti because I wanted to make a difference in other people's lives. At the same time, I thought to myself: 'If I can go over there and help them, it'll be one of those feelings where I've been able to help somebody, but they can never repay me.'

I was so mistaken, because the joy that they brought into my life far outweighs the joy that I've brought into theirs. My time in Haiti had only just begun, because my life changed forever when I trekked back from that mountain.

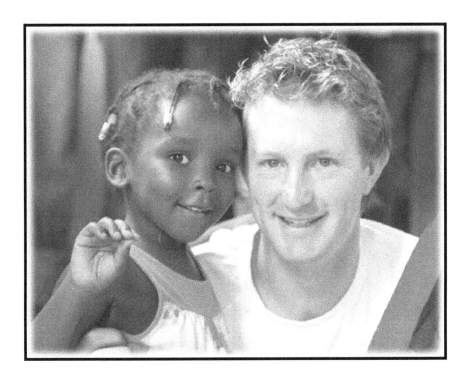

My 'favourite' little angel in my orphanage in Haiti, 2013.

On our way back down the mountain before heading home to Australia, we arrived at an 'orphanage'. (It was really a heartbreaking open-air compound with torn tarps for makeshift walls.) There were 20 little kids, and they had no clothes, no food, and no shelter, but they all had one thing in common: astoundingly, they all had a smile on their face. These kids had nothing. They had no mum or dad. They had lost everything in the earthquake. Yet, they still had life. They still had dreams. They still had hope for a brighter future.

It was something that has helped me become the person I am today, because it put so many things into perspective. I asked one little boy the best part about being there, and he commented that he gets a bowl of rice every other day. The worst part was the fact that he had to share a bed with two little boys who both still pee their pants, and they all got soaking wet at night.

In my life, I spend so much time on the roads and in hotels. Sometimes I complain about the hotels where I am staying. I walk into the room, I see 10 pillows on the bed, and I think to myself: 'What do I need with 10 pillows? I only need one.' After I remove nine pillows, I go to climb into bed, and I think that the cleaner must think that I am a cardboard cut-out; they tuck the sheets in so flipping tight that you need to rip out the sheets just so you can get into the bed. Then, your feet are so squashed at the end of the bed that they feel like flippers.

How dare I complain: These guys are not complaining because the roof leaks, because they have no family, and that little boy is not complaining that he is getting peed on. These kids are celebrating each day the mere fact that they are alive; they are breathing. They count their blessings every day, not their problems.

The happiest people don't have the best of everything; they just make the best of everything. I think to myself throughout these hard times and challenging moments that 'A star does not shine without darkness'. These angels are certainly shining in my heart.

The plight of the people of Haiti tore out my heart, and I really felt I needed to do more. My friends and I went back to Australia, and we raised a whole heap of money. Then, a dear friend of mine, Simon O'Dell, and I got on a plane and ventured back to Haiti together in order to rebuild the orphanage from the ground up.

I remember the first day I was there. We were exhausted. We were lying in a tiny concrete shack, and it was overwhelming: the heat, the noise, the smell, the mosquitoes, the uncomfortable bed, with just a tiny fan on the end of my bed to keep me cool. There was a generator outside, constantly roaring, making a horrible racket. I got next to no sleep, and I had to film for the documentary *Hope for Haiti* the very next morning.

I remember waking up and saying to the man who was running that area: 'Why, why, did you need that generator going all night? The bed was uncomfortable. The mosquitoes were biting me. The noise was horrendous. The temperature was brutal.'

He said to me: 'Michael, I'm sorry, I can't do anything about the heat. Nor can I do anything about the comfort of your bed, or the mosquitoes.' He added: 'And I'm sorry about the noise from the generator, but I had one of the young orphans sleep on the roof, where the generator sits, and he topped up the generator with fuel, every two hours, to make sure that we had enough power to run the fan on the end of your bed.'

Sometimes it's so powerful when you step out of your own shoes and look at life through someone else's eyes. You quickly begin to realise that your problems, your challenges, your adversity, your pain, and your suffering can be so insignificant in comparison to the struggles of people who live in developing nations.

The next two weeks were the hardest and the most emotionally draining of the trip, but they were the most rewarding experience of my life. There was not one day on the work site where we felt alone.

There was not one day where there wasn't a seven-year-old boy, with no mum or dad or brothers or sisters, with a hammer in his hand, and a nail, ready to do whatever it took to help.

I remember that one day Simon and I went down to buy the beds — the new beds that these kids were going to sleep in. So many of them were just lying on pieces of tin, timber or steel. The first shop we went into, we found that the mattresses were $100 each. When Simon and I walked into pay, they quickly increased that amount to $380 per mattress.

We had only been funded $2000 for 20 mattresses. There was no way in the world that we were going to be able to afford it. We had to go to other stores, stay on the back of the truck, and let the guys from the orphanage go in to pay for it to prevent us from being ripped off.

We had a security guard, Samuel, who stayed on the edge of the truck with us the whole time. After purchasing the mattresses, he left the truck to go in to get the mattresses. Talk about fear and anxiety!

We were in this scary place, where people wanted a piece of us because we weren't helping them. The truck started to be surrounded by people, and not nice people; they were people who had machetes, and who wanted our money.

They were people who wanted us to help *them*, not help the people we were helping. Fortunately enough, our prayers were answered: when Samuel and the rest of the team came running out with mattresses, they all ran off, so we were OK.

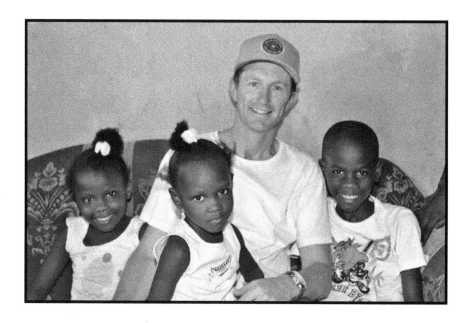

Spending some relaxation time with the kids in Haiti after rebuilding the orphanage.

We went back to the orphanage with all of our gear, and we transformed the orphanage from a run-down, old tin shack to somewhere that these kids could call home. We turned it into something that these kids were proud of. They helped paint the walls. They helped put the beds together. They helped create something that was special to them.

There have been plenty of memories of my time in Haiti. Good memories, bad memories, sad and emotional memories, but I continue to reflect on why I went there in the first place. I went there because I wanted to make a difference in someone's life, where they could never, ever make a difference in mine. Surprise! They made more of a difference in mine than I could ever make in theirs.

Nine months later, I was fortunate to get on the plane to head back over there with a very dear friend of mine, Wayne Glenn, a member of the Coffs Harbour Rotary Team. Very sadly, Wayne passed away in 2015.

We went over there to put a second storey on the orphanage, and to put new beds and more mattresses in there. We also built them a kitchen, a toilet and a shower. When they first saw the toilet, these kids had no idea what to do. They thought it was a basin to drink out of. It really smacks you in the face when you need to educate a 10-year-old boy on how to use a toilet, because they've never seen one before.

The people in the church and community surrounding the orphanage have a heart for giving. They would give you the last dime they had. They would give you the last piece of food they had. They would take the clothes off their back for you, to provide for you.

It's interesting to see so many videos nowadays online, where a homeless man will go up and ask a very wealthy man who is eating a pizza whether he can have a piece, and the wealthy man replies: 'No.'

They will ask a wealthy lady who gets change from her purchase at Myer whether they could borrow a dollar, and she'll reply, 'No.' Then, they give a homeless man a pizza, and another man will walk past and ask: 'Is there any chance I could have a piece of pizza?', and the homeless man quickly gives him half of his pizza.

Why is it that the more we gain in life, the more we expect? But, when we lose everything, it's almost like our outlook completely changes, and we realise that giving is so much more powerful and so much more rewarding than receiving.

My journey of compassion and love for the country of Haiti still continues to this day. I truly believe in my heart that Haiti's people have changed my life forever. They have taught me some really powerful and life-changing lessons that I am forever grateful for: they have taught me that when you change the way you look at things, the things you look at change. These kids have nothing: no family, no laptops or iPhones, but they wake up each morning and think they have everything. And the reason they believe that is because they woke up that morning.

I regularly think to myself, 'Can you imagine if that was the way the entire world worked? Can you imagine if each and every one of us got out of bed every morning and were truly grateful because we got out of bed this morning?' If we believed in ourselves and realised that we could overcome any challenge, any heartache, any pain, any suffering that this world might throw at us, because we had the incredible blessing of getting out of bed this morning?

I try and live my life by the saying, 'We must give without remembering and receive without forgetting'. I think that when we begin to live our life with this motto, it is only then we begin to discover how blessed we are to have what we have.

I still go to Haiti three or four times a year to see how I can add value and continue to bring peace and happiness to these wonderful kids. What's been an incredible discovery over the last 12 to 18 months is that we have begun to realise that, out of the 40-plus children who now live in the orphanage, over 16 of them have parents who are still alive.

We have worked on a program to reintroduce these kids, many of whom believed that their parents had died. Many of the parents had also thought their children had died, but, as I'm sure you can imagine, unfortunately, several of the parents gave their kids away because they could no longer take care of them.

So now we are in the process of reintroducing these beautiful kids to their families. And I have never been so overwhelmed and emotionally fuelled as by this interaction. Can you imagine — just for a moment — that eight or nine years ago you believed that your child had passed away, and then all of a sudden someone comes knocking on your door to inform you that that is not the case?

Unfortunately, many of the parents live below the poverty line — they do not work, they have no home, they live in tent cities — so we are unable to return these kids to their parents. As you can image, the emotional roller-coaster ride for these parents would be significant, discovering that their children are still alive and then not being able to take them back.

So we have been working on a program, to teach the parents how to fish. We have built a training and development centre for these parents, under four different pillars: construction, English speaking, sewing and also jewellery making. We have now been able to help these parents set up their own micro businesses, allowing them to be in control of their future. And now we have been able to reintroduce many of these kids, and place them back into their family's home. And if the family doesn't have a home, we are also trying to help these families get one, so that they can be together as one united family after all this heartache and pain.

We know that the best place for a child is to be with their family. And we will do everything we can to try and find a place for each of these beautiful children to live.

Sadly, in late 2019 there was a coup in Haiti where everything was closed — shops, hospitals, you name it — and sadly one of the beautiful boys from our orphanage got sick and we could not get him treatment anywhere. He passed away at the age of 11. It was obviously heartbreaking for everybody involved, not only the kids in the orphanage, but also the team at Frontier Projects who work tirelessly to support these kids, and also the sponsor, a very dear friend of mine, who lives in Melbourne. He said to me that it was like he lost one of his own children.

Which just demonstrates so beautifully the power of giving and the impact that we can have when we have a passion to simply serve other people, expecting nothing in return.

OPTIMISM &
RESILIENCE
HELP YOU NOT JUST
SURVIVE
BUT THRIVE
THROUGH
UNCERTAIN
TIMES.

(12)

A DREAM FOLLOWED
BY A NIGHTMARE

I was already passionate about the power of giving, but one of the greatest days of my life came when I finally got a chance to give something to someone who has sacrificed so much for me. It was the day I put a pink ribbon on the door of a new home for my mum to live the rest of her life in. I will never forget the tears in her eyes and the smile that she had in her heart. She was glowing with pride and joy. The feeling of happiness is so much greater when you give as opposed to when you receive. Sure, the money that comes out of my account each week to pay the mortgage is not fun, however what is fun is the sense of pride in knowing I have been able to give back. That was the day where I finally could look at myself in the mirror and be proud of who I had become.

Two weeks after that amazing day, unfortunately, my wife convinced me that there was something wrong. She had noticed a lump in my throat. I didn't think anything of it until she said that it looked like I had another Adam's apple. I underwent test after test, and was poked, prodded, X-rayed and scanned. During that time, I couldn't help but allow my mind to wander. One night I dreamed about what the doctors might say, and I got into the shower to try to clear my mind because I had almost convinced myself that the doctors were going to tell me that the lump was a terminal cancer. I immediately vomited in the shower and I felt like I was going to pass out. I think in that instant I really began to understand the power of my mind. I realised that if I did not control it and have it in the best possible place, my life could become a real mess.

The support that I have from my family, friends and social media followers is, at times, extremely overwhelming, and I certainly feel very blessed to have these wonderful people in my life.

I've begun to realise that it is the people who are around the challenge who hurt more than the person who is actually dealing with it. I've begun to understand by watching my mum deal with her emotional challenges that the people surrounding the sick actually hurt more, because these are the people who truly have no control. And I think that when you are out of control, you find it very difficult to deal with that situation.

Throughout all those years when Mum would receive my test results, her response to me was always the same: 'Son, everything will be OK.' But she knew deep down inside that was not the case. She carried that burden and the pain so I didn't need to. It's amazing the sacrifices that some people in this world make to support other people's physical and emotional needs. I think that is why I love that song, 'People helping people', because I regularly think to myself: can you imagine if every single day every single one of us got out of bed and had a dream and a goal to simply just help people? I truly believe that it would be heaven on earth.

I finally received the phone call that my results were in. I went in and sat down with the doctor, and he told me the news that I was so fearful of for such a long time. I remember his words so clearly. He said to me, 'Unfortunately Michael, we have not just found one lump, but rather we have found four tumours in your throat. Your tomorrows aren't guaranteed, and you need to slow down.' I remember replying without really even thinking or digesting what he'd said, 'That is one thing that we all have in common.' None of us are guaranteed tomorrow.

And that's why I truly believe that we must live in the present moment and embrace every opportunity and every day as a gift, a bonus, and a blessing because that is exactly what it is. I walked out of the doctor's office and my phone rang; it was my mum. I knew exactly what she was going to ask me and I knew exactly what I was going to say. She said to me, 'Son, what did the doctor say?' And I finally got to return the favour. I told my mum, 'Everything will be OK.'

I returned home; I hadn't spoken to my wife yet because she was at work. And I got into the shower and I vomited in fear. I was about to get myself into bed and have a big pity party when I realised that I had to do something. I had to get my mind cleared, my heart racing. Something I'd begun to realise over many years, but implemented on this day, was that to shift our mindset, to get above the line, to be a pilot and not a passenger, to be a navigator and not a victim, we must do three simple things:

1. move

2. share

3. help.

I got in the car and I drove down to the beach and went for a run on the sand to get my mind clear, my heart racing and the endorphins flowing.

Regardless of our age or gender, we all benefit from increased activity, from doing something, anything — the health benefits are hard to ignore. Going for a walk, a run, anything that increases your blood flow will ultimately give you more energy and make you feel better.

When you engage in physical activity you burn calories. The more intense the activity, the more calories you burn. Regular trips to the gym are great, but don't worry if you can't find a large chunk of time to exercise every day. Any amount of activity is better than none at all. Take the stairs instead of the elevator, do some laps instead of just sunbaking, ride the bike instead of catching the bus or even get off one stop early on your normal bus route home. All you need is a heart starter, 20 minutes a day ...

Increased activity will also help prevent or manage a wide range of health problems and concerns, including stroke, high blood pressure, Type 2 diabetes, depression, anxiety, many types of cancer and even arthritis.

I like to think I am Mr Positive, but sometimes I find myself in need of a little emotional lift or desperate to blow off some steam after a stressful day. A run or walk amongst nature can change everything. What's amazing is that if you force yourself to do it, even though you don't feel like it, you ultimately feel so much better for the activity, and will always end up thanking yourself for it. The morning is the ideal time to set you up for a powerful day: it's better for weight loss, metabolism, and it means it's done!

Physical activity, it doesn't matter what type, will stimulate various brain chemicals, which in turn trigger a feeling of happiness and ultimately leave you feeling more relaxed and less anxious. You may also feel better about your appearance and yourself when you exercise, which also has the added advantage of boosting your confidence and improving your self-esteem.

What I find amazing is how moving creates energy even when you're flat. Moving or exercising delivers oxygen and nutrients to your tissues and helps your cardiovascular system work more efficiently. The net result of improved heart and lung health is the creation of more energy.

Being on the road all the time, I sometimes really struggle to sleep. Experience has proven to me that I enjoy a much sounder and more restful sleep if I increase my level of physical activity during the day. Physical activity helps me slow my brain down, and I don't go to bed with my mind racing, which of course is counterproductive to a good night's sleep.

I also believe that moving regularly during the day has a direct correlation to an improved sex life. At the risk of sharing too much information, I find that when I don't go out and do something and instead spend the day lounging around on the couch feeling sorry for myself, I don't even feel as though I have the energy to enjoy physical intimacy. Conversely, when I get out into the fresh air and get the heart pumping, my endorphins start to flow, and everything is more positive.

Moving and regular activity has the added advantage of bringing something very important into your life — connection with people! Not only does it give you a chance to unwind and enjoy the outdoors, it also provides the opportunity to connect with family or friends in a fun, social setting. Friends can fuel the heart, and sometimes when we are a little flat, that is all we really need to get moving and bring a smile to our face.

Physical activity contributes to a feeling of wellbeing. Increased movement will boost your health, it will assist in shifting your mindset and will help take you away from what is holding you back or weighing you down.

* * *

Let's return to my run on the beach after I found out about the tumours in my throat. While on the run I ran into a dear friend of mine, Clint Greenshields, a former NRL superstar, and we got chatting for an extended period of time. I realised this was my moment to share; this was an opportunity for me to get things off my chest. I was beginning to realise it was not a sign of weakness, but rather a sign of strength. This was the second step: sharing.

When we realise the importance of seeking help and sharing our challenges, our pain and our suffering with a peer, a colleague, a friend, a coach or even a counsellor, I think it's actually the first step in our transformation, and an important step in healing the pain.

If we are serious about wanting to regain control of our life, improve our level of happiness and redirect our mindset, we must reach out and connect with the people who are important to us. We must communicate, get our problems off our chest, and seek some clarity and direction.

I believe the key to any great relationship is the ability to effectively communicate, and sometimes we simply need to free our brain from emotional overload. We need to get things out of our crazy, fast-paced minds and create space for calmness and, ultimately, enjoyment. Sharing how you feel and what you are going through with a peer or a friend or a counsellor is very therapeutic. Putting your hand up and asking for help may not be the easiest thing to do — in fact, quite the opposite — but I believe it shows a strength of character, a determination and a desire to turn things around in your life, that is courageous and to be admired.

There is no doubt that we all have problems in our life from time to time. Some problems may feel tolerable, whereas others feel overwhelming and unmanageable. Regardless of the intensity, severity and frequency of your problem, no issue is too small or too big to benefit from sharing with friends, family or a professional. A problem shared is a problem halved, and with practice being vulnerable, it's a game changer: it builds trust in a personal and professional environment. It's not weakness; it actually shows strength and character.

Friends and family can be great sources of support, however in some cases they can be quick to give advice and often dive right into 'fix it' mode. How often have we heard statements such as, 'Well, that happened to me and I did X, Y and Z ... You really should try that, it worked for me'? When this happens, the focus of the conversation is shifted away from you and your unique experience. Their advice is from their viewpoint, which may not resonate with you or apply to your specific situation.

Prioritising your mental health promotes healthy self-care practices, and, just as you take care of your physical health, it is equally important to take care of your mental health. It is for this reason that sharing your thoughts and feelings, when they become too heavy or overwhelming, with a counsellor or other professional can be a huge step in the right direction. Everyone needs an outlet, ideally a mental health professional with whom they can unload all the 'heavy stuff'. Talking about your problems without censoring any of the sensitive details can be liberating!

When our problems become overwhelming it is very common to ask the question 'Why is this happening to me?' It is natural to want to know the reasons and, in many cases, understanding these reasons can set the parameters for our recovery. Therapy is a process that can help you better understand yourself and provide you with new coping strategies to manage current and future problems. Therefore, I believe that, regardless of the problem, the type of stress or hardship, everyone can benefit from seeking the help and support of a counsellor or other professional. I have also realised that a great first step to 'sharing', if you're not comfortable with speaking to someone else yet, is to try a little journalling. Downloading your thoughts in a journal can help massively in releasing tension and gaining clarity, and will help you get laser focused. The one and only key when journalling is simple: start each sentence with 'I feel'.

Regular check-ups are as important for us as they are for our cars. It seems crazy that we will go to the expense of getting our car serviced, but we won't take the time to check up on our own physical and mental wellbeing. We all know that regardless of how great our car's shiny new rims are, how amazing the paintwork looks or how awesome the sunroof and leather seats are, if the engine doesn't work, we are not going anywhere. Similarly, we can get into shape physically, get a six-pack and tone our body, get our hair and make-up looking on point, but if we can't get our brain, our emotions and our mental approach to life right, then, just like that car, we're not going anywhere. Remember, we are human beings and not human doings — that's the power of sharing.

* * *

Finally, the last of these three steps was about helping someone else. After sharing what I was going through with Clint on the beach, he invited me back to his house and we had dinner, and Mel joined us. I really like to help people, so on my way home from having dinner I stopped at the service station and filled my car up with fuel. When I went inside I paid for my fuel, bowser seven, and then I paid for the fuel on bowser eight. I got in the car and I was about to drive off and I thought, 'No, no, I'll wait and I'll see that lady when she goes in to pay for bowser eight and realises that it's paid for.' She went in to pay, and I could see the gentleman behind the counter gesture towards me. I remember her looking out at me. She smiled and mouthed 'thank you' and I drove off.

I felt great for a moment. But then I realised the only reason I had done something for her was to get something in return — and that was to have her thank me.

So now when I pay for other people's fuel, I drive off without them knowing and that makes me feel even better. Because I'm doing it just to make an impact on somebody else, not to be thanked for serving someone else.

Scientists have been studying a phenomenon called 'helper's high', testing the theory that helping others releases endorphins which, in turn, improves mood and boosts self-esteem. In fact, it is possible that helping others does more for the happiness of the person helping than the person who receives the help.

I have come to realise over the years that it feels far greater to give than to receive, as does it feel greater to help than to be helped. I believe that when I help someone in need it gives me an endorphin hit; it makes me feel good about myself and it makes me feel personally valued as a quality human being.

The personal happiness gained by undertaking random acts of kindness can become addictive and can see you striving daily to identify people and situations where you can lend a hand, where you can bring happiness to people and in turn create a smile in your own heart. As I've said before, one of my favourite sayings is 'We must give without remembering and receive without forgetting'. Sadly, in too many cases, the world we live in today works with the opposite mentality.

I have spent a great deal of time thinking about the many different ways I can help people on a daily basis and make a positive impact on their day. This focus has come as a result of hearing too many people suggest that they will be happy to spend more time helping others in the future, when they are richer or in a better financial position. So I've been focusing on what I can do to help people and make an impact on their life now, but without requiring me spending any money. Just yesterday I was walking along the footpath when I noticed a lady opening her car to start unloading a very large shopping trolley full of groceries. I said to her, 'Do you mind if I help you unpack your shopping?'

To which she replied, 'Oh my, thanks so much — aren't you all about acts of kindness?'

We chatted, laughed and she even gave me a hug as I left. I walked away feeling a little taller, with my chest puffed out, knowing that I had just in a very small way made that lady feel special. For all I know that may have been the only piece of kindness that she would receive that day, but it may just help shift her mindset and have her realise that there are still kind people in the world. It was a win-win as we both felt better after the very simple encounter. As I waked away, an elderly gentleman smiled at me and said, 'You've made that lady's day, young fella, and you've also made me smile.' It was a win-win-win!

The link between better health and helping others is striking. Studies prove that if you want to live longer you need to be a helper/giver. According to these studies, helping or giving to others has a positive impact on our mental health. Current research is very careful not to draw too many conclusions as to the reasons why, but I believe that simply making positive contact with others improves our positive feelings about ourselves.

Humans are basically hardwired for social interactions. Interactions such as touch, eye contact and even smiling release oxytocin, a chemical that helps us manage stress and ultimately results in a happier, healthier us.

The idea that there is a link between a meaningful life and helping others is actually a rather old one. Carol Ryff is an American academic and psychologist who is known for studying psychological wellbeing and resilience. Carol Ryff's Model of Psychological Well-being outlines six criteria, including self-acceptance, personal growth, purpose in life and positive relations with others. The overarching constant in all the criteria is that helping others is a central feature of a positive, well-lived and meaningful life.

I'm sure you've heard of 'paying it forward'. We do things to make an impact on others in the hope not of something in return, but rather the hope for a ripple effect in creating a greater impact than we thought possible.

Here are some simple ways to help others that cost you nothing:

- ask the people you deal with on a daily basis what you could do to make their jobs easier

- push a stranger's shopping trolley to their car for them (after asking for permission)

- return trolleys to the trolley bay (even abandoned ones)

- businesspeople or frequent travellers: use your frequent flier status to help another traveller into the lounge for a free lunch or coffee or just space to relax

- offer your help whenever and wherever possible

- donate your time and your skills wherever needed

- donate your time with charity events/fundraisers/school barbecues/community groups

- pick up some rubbish that is not yours

- mow your neighbour's lawn

- tidy your home and gift your old toys and clothes to people in need

- blow dry your partner's hair

- surprise your partner with getting some chores done around the home.

The expectations you walk past are the expectations you set. Do acts of kindness as though the whole world is watching, even if no-one really is. Doing these things will shift your mindset and have you hungry to identify more opportunities every day to help more people. A meaningful life isn't found, but created through our actions, and it starts with looking for ways to help others and act in a way that would make your future self proud.

* * *

So those were my three steps. I had to move, I had to share and I had to help.

When I arrived home after paying for the woman's fuel, my wife said to me, 'Oh and how did you go today at the doctors?' I thought to myself, 'What would my response have been if I hadn't moved, shared and helped? What would my response have been if I had just called her and told her exactly the words?' And, 'What would the outcome have been if I'd have sat around in a pity party and believed that my life wasn't fair and that I wasn't going to make it?'

I told Mel, 'They've found some tumours in my throat. It's going to be a battle, but with you by my side, I know in my heart that everything will be OK.'

It's remarkable: when we shift our mindset the outcome can be tremendous. And I truly believe that shifting my mindset could possibly have saved my life.

WHEN WE STRIVE TO SERVE $ NOT EARN WE TRULY FIND OUR PURPOSE.

13

STRIVING TO SERVE, NOT EARN

The surgery was all booked in. And yes, there was a sense of anxiety and fear, without a doubt. But I needed to have faith and confidence knowing that everything was going to be okay. Still, I really wanted to make sure that I spent some quality time with my wife before I went into surgery. I had an amazing dinner with my family a week before the surgery. I gave them all a hug and a kiss and told them how much I loved them.

The morning before we got in the car to drive up to Brisbane I did a video message saying goodbye to my family. I wanted to make sure that if I wasn't to make it through the surgery that everybody knew exactly how I felt about them. How much I loved them. How grateful I was for the impact that they had on my life. And I think too often we wait until it's too late before we decide to share with those around us how much they mean to us. I made sure that if I was to pass away there was no uncertainty. And also that my funeral was all covered, because I didn't want my family to have to worry about any of that.

So we drove to Brisbane and we stopped off at Hope Island, where Mel and I hired a houseboat for five days to be away from the world. No social media, no interaction with anybody else; just a really special moment and a remarkable opportunity for my wife and I to simply be present. To be together with no distractions. Because my outlook on life is that the quality of one's life is not dictated or determined by the amount of days that we live on this earth. Rather, it's what we fit into those days that allows us to live a remarkable life.

I wanted this moment to be really special. To be together. To be truly present. To show one another the love that we have. And I also wanted her to have nothing but beautiful memories. If these were the last times we spent together.

The boat trip was amazing. We had the most beautiful weather. The water was spectacular. We played games, we laughed, we giggled, we hugged and we cried. But we were together. The last night on the boat was crazy; it was almost like a sign from above. We were radioed from the houseboat office telling us that there was a huge storm rolling in and that we needed to head back to the office. However, we were so far away we wouldn't have made it back before dark, and houseboats can't travel at night. So they told us what we must do. We needed to open all the zippers upstairs. We needed to lay all the furniture down. We needed to extend the anchor rope so that the boat had a little bit of flex.

And then I came up with this genius idea: if we went to bed early and tried to fall asleep before the storm hit, then maybe we'd wake up in the morning not having even noticed the storm! So we got into bed nice and early, I put my earplugs in and off to sleep I went. It was almost the best sleep I'd ever had.

I woke up the next morning, fresh and ready to take on the day. I looked over at Mel and said, 'That storm didn't even hit. I feel so good and I'm ready.'

She looked at me and rolled her eyes and said she'd got maybe two hours of sleep because the storm had hit and she was up all night trying to hold down the furniture, making sure the boat was facing the right way and ensuring that nothing went overboard. I had slept through the entire storm. Clearly I'd needed the rest!

We got back to the office and dropped the boat off, then we got in the car and drove up to Brisbane. We arrived at Brisbane Private Hospital nice and early, ready to go to battle. And then I heard the words, 'Michael, it's time to come through.' I gave my beautiful wife a hug and a kiss and walked through those doors. It was only once I had got through those doors that I realised that that hug and that kiss may have been the very last ones I ever got to give my wife.

They told Mel that I would be out in about three hours if everything went to plan. I can only imagine the fear that she

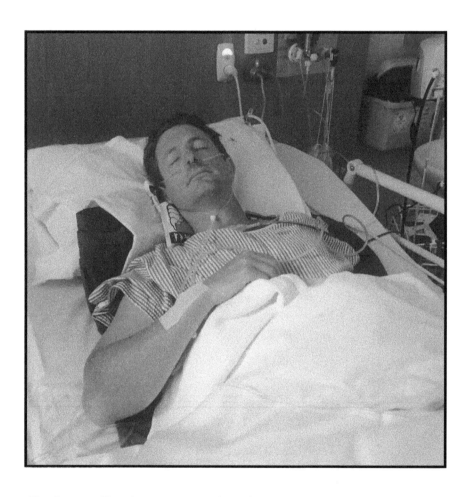

The photo my wife took post-surgery to share with everyone that I was out and breathing.

must have felt sitting in that waiting room, hoping and praying that her husband came out alive. Two hours passed. Three hours passed. Four, five hours, six hours had passed, and I still hadn't returned. She was having a meltdown. Eventually someone came out and told her that my surgery had been delayed by three hours due to a backlog. So, they were expecting me out in about an hour.

Finally, I came through. I remember waking up and seeing my beautiful wife. She was holding my hand letting me know that everything was OK.

As I write this, the tears flow down my face. Not tears of sadness, but rather tears of complete and utter gratitude. Not only for the medical professionals for helping once again to save my life, but, just as important, to have the love of my life holding my hand with complete love and faith in knowing that everything was going to be OK.

The surgeon came in (and I must say he looked like he was about 20), and he said, 'Surgery was partly a success.' Which obviously had us a little puzzled. He went on to tell us that they had removed three out of the four tumours. The fourth tumour is benign — it could possibly stay in my throat for the rest of my life and not give me any grief at all — and it is tangled up with my vocal cords, so removing it would almost certainly leave me unable to speak. However, it could grow and that would require immediate surgery. So every 90 days I go in and get checked to make sure there has been no growth.

For me, the surgery was a huge success, because I was still here, I was still smiling, and I was still breathing. They weren't certain of the impact, if any, it had had on my vocal cords. But they did ask me not to say anything for three days. I think Mel was over the moon; she loved the peace and serenity. But after three days I was finally allowed to try and use my vocal cords, and I could speak. The first few words that I whispered were to my wife, telling her that I loved her.

Reflecting on these words, it makes me realise how lucky I am to still be here, but also how important it is to share your heart and your soul with people. To give them your honesty, your empathy, and have them understand exactly how you feel about them. I think when we live a life free of regrets, that's when we start to live our life on purpose.

I was told to probably take six weeks off for the surgery, to allow myself to heal. But I had other ideas. I was feeling great, I was feeling positive, I was feeling clear and excited about my future. And 19 days later I stepped on stage, in front of over 1000 people at a national conference in Perth, feeling as though I could take on the world. I shared my journey and the success of the surgery with them, and all the while I had no idea how my world was about to change.

* * *

As I have previously mentioned, the transition out of the corporate world and doing my best to make it in the speaking world was not easy. But I think nothing that's worthwhile is easy. I think for quite a while I was speaking to earn a living.

But when I started to speak purely to make an impact as my number one priority, then everything changed. Not only the delivery and the messaging, but the *why* behind every time I got on stage. I clearly remember saying to Mel one day, 'If I ever get on stage just simply to earn an income, that is the day I will stop speaking on stage forever.'

It's amazing: in the speaking world people want to be on stage in front of 20 000 people and getting paid a fortune before they've earned their stripes, before they've pounded the pavement, before they've had a million 'noes' before they finally get that one 'yes'. And I think that that's what I needed to do. I needed to learn to take every single event, every single opportunity, to see myself and my career and my profile grow. And it's amazing how my profile and my career drastically transformed from an event that I was not even being paid to speak at.

It all began when I started to do more and more talks for Camp Quality. The more events I did for them, the more exposure I got to different companies. I was speaking at one event, and the CEO of 7-Eleven was there. He said to me after my presentation, 'Michael, I want you to speak at my company conference.'

I thought it might have been another one of those 'offer you the world, deliver you nothing' situations, but it was quite the opposite. We formed a wonderful friendship and, in fact, when I spoke for his company I stayed at his beautiful home in Melbourne. After speaking at that event he told me that he wanted me to speak at another conference, which was how I found out that he was actually one of the major sponsors at the HR Forum, a huge annual event attended by all the decision makers from all the big companies across the country. He had asked them to have me speak, but because my profile wasn't big enough and they had no idea who I was, they declined.

He went back to them and said, 'Well if you want my sponsorship money you will have Michael speak at this conference. And we'd like him to speak last.' They save the last spot for the best speaker, and because I was not on their radar they said, 'Not a chance.' However, they agreed to have me as the second last speaker.

Obviously, I was very excited. I went along to this very large conference not knowing that off the back of this event my speaking career was going to change. I spoke at this event in front of over 1000 people, and it was the first standing ovation that group had ever given in 20-plus years. All of a sudden my emails started to go crazy, my calendar started to fill up and the roller-coaster of speaking in the professional world had certainly begun. But what I realised after that event is when you're getting paid to speak it doesn't necessarily mean that you've made it — and it doesn't necessarily mean that you're in the right place.

I got asked to do an event in Los Angeles and I had my agent ask what was their budget. They said they had no budget, but there was a part of my heart that said I still needed to do this.

So I went to Los Angeles, and I did the event — but I hadn't realised I was going to share the stage with the likes of the Dalai Lama, Kelly Slater and Tony Hawk. And I didn't realise that there were going to be people in the audience who were going to be very, very influential and were going to change my life forever.

There is a gentleman in the United States by the name of Rob Dyrdek. He is the host of an MTV show called *Ridiculousness*, which I must say is one of my favourite shows because it takes me away from what might be happening in my world and allows me to just laugh until my stomach gets sore. It's a show that compiles viral videos from around the world, with the hosts adding hilarious commentary, and there are some interviews thrown in for good measure. He said to me, 'Mike, I really love your story, your presentation and I would really love to have you on my show.' As you can imagine, I went ballistic — I was just so excited. But once again I had that reserve in me, thinking this could be just another one of those situations.

I flew back to Australia and unfortunately I never heard from him again ... or so I thought. Because five months later I received a phone call from a producer of *Ridiculousness* telling me that Rob had finally found a time slot and they were going to fly me over to the United States — up the front of the plane, which was amazing — to film my episode. I remember telling my friends and my family that it was going to be incredible and I was so excited.

They put me up in this beautiful hotel in Beverley Hills and I had no idea when I arrived that there was going to be paparazzi everywhere. I arrived in a huge black Escalade and all these guys were standing around with their cameras, waiting to take photos. I didn't realise that Justin Bieber, Jerry Springer and Phil Collins were also staying in the same hotel.

I got out of the car with my big hat and sunglasses on, feeling like a celebrity. They all looked up with their cameras...then realised that I was a nobody and put the cameras straight back down. I went into my fancy room and got over my jet lag, and two days later the driver was there ready to take me to the studio. When I arrived I had goosebumps all over me. I was so, so excited.

The show was one of the most amazing experiences. So much fun, so much laughter, so much joy and happiness — and the episode of mine, which was aired directly after it was filmed, was a huge success. It was viewed by millions and millions of people around the world. They still to this day repeat my episode and it's something that I'm very proud of — and it was a lot of fun.

After filming the show, I was at the business lounge in Los Angeles. A guy by the name of Paul Worsteling, who is the host of a TV show called *IFISH*, approached me and said, 'I just saw you on *Ridiculousness*. I loved your show. Is there a chance I could get you on my show?' Long story short, I was lucky enough to be invited to be on the season finale of his fishing show. We went to an incredible place called Cobourg Peninsula, up past Darwin. We fished for five days to produce what I thought was going to be one episode.

However, the fishing was so insane up there we had a one-hour season finale plus four 30-minute episodes. And I'm not a fisherman, so that shows you how good the fishing was.

In fact, the fishing was so crazy that at one stage I had caught a fish and had taken it off the hook (or to be more accurate, Paul took it off the hook) and, as we turned to do a piece to camera, I lobbed the lure over the side of the boat again. A fish jumped out of the water and immediately grabbed the lure. It was like shooting fish in a barrel — they were absolutely everywhere.

So my profile started to grow. My social media online presence started to increase. And then I was asked by an online platform, called Gold Cast, whether I would be open to them editing one of my presentations and sharing it online. I said, 'Sure, I would love that.' I didn't realise that that video was going to go viral! And that there were going to be some overwhelmingly positive, but also negative, things that occurred off the back of it.

I remember the day the video, titled 'How to fight through the worst of times' was launched online: within two hours it got over 100 000 views, and I remember saying to Mel, 'Oh my God, this video is going crazy. Can you imagine if we got to like half a million views?' That afternoon we checked and it'd already got up to 480 000 views — we were over the moon.

When we woke up the next morning it had over a million views. This video had been online for less than 24 hours and it already had a million views. Fast forward to now and that video has been viewed by more than 60 million people around the world.

That obviously massively opened up my global reach and allowed me to have some remarkable opportunities to travel the world and share my story. That video was viewed by the likes of Sir Richard Branson, who invited me to speak on his stage for his Australian tour in late 2019. And then I was asked to speak at none other than Tony Robbins' Australian tour in 2020. The messages that I received were overwhelming. And I was really flying on cloud 9.

However, unfortunately, in this world there is very much a tall poppy syndrome, where some people do their absolute best to bring you down when they see you succeeding. I experienced some incredible online bullying from trolls who didn't like to see an ordinary old Australian succeeding in the world. What was amazing was my mindset was incredibly challenged by these people. I would wake up in the morning and I would have over 1000 messages. I would start to read through the messages, from people who don't know who I am but have just seen a video of mine. And 999 of them might be super positive, about how much it's changed their outlook and their life and their relationships and their health. But I'd read one that was negative — I couldn't help myself — and all of a sudden my mind, and my body and my soul, everything was channelled into that one negative person who said those negative words.

Through this experience I came to realise a couple of things. Firstly, your value does not decrease based on a random person's inability to see your worth. I think that it is so incredibly important that we understand who we are, and the value that we bring to the world. We can't allow other people's uneducated opinions of us to dictate what type of life we get to live. I think too often we allow the negativity of other people to cripple us and steer us down a path that doesn't allow us to become the best version of ourselves.

And I try and remember to not take criticism from those you would not take advice from. That for me has been a really powerful lesson that I continue to reflect on daily. I understand the importance of believing in me, believing in what I stand for and knowing that my passion and my purpose is to simply get out of bed and make a difference in just one person's life. It is so remarkable what we can achieve by simply believing in ourselves, and not putting any limited beliefs within our own hearts. While I'm only human and I still get challenged emotionally and mentally to get through that environment of doubt and fear and anxiety, I reflect constantly on ensuring that I'm doing everything that I possibly can to mentally be in a great place.

In late 2019 I was asked to speak at an event in Kansas City. It was very, very cold. I got there three days before the event and I was asked to keep a low profile and avoid being seen by people in the hotel, because I was the big surprise. (I must say it was probably unnecessary, as many of them probably had no idea who I was.) But I needed to make sure that I stayed out of sight because they had booked the entire hotel.

So I basically spent three days in the hotel wishing that I was at home. And I started to question why I was doing this: being on the road for eight months a year. Being away from the people I loved and those who loved me. But then I began to realise we must understand what recharges our batteries. What actually allows us to stay in control. And yes, I've spoken about it before: we must move, share and help to get through those dark times.

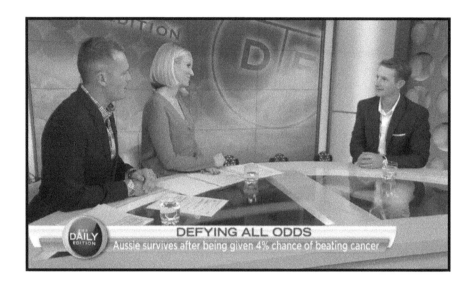

DEFYING ALL ODDS
Aussie survives after being given 4% chance of beating cancer

Sharing my journey on The Daily Edition TV show.

On the Studio 10 TV show, letting the country know Mel and I were expecting a baby.

But what recharges us? I realised that night in that hotel room that if I was to just turn my phone off at night and leave it unplugged, then the next morning the phone would still operate, but it would not have recharged. And that's similar to us: I believe that we go to bed, we have a good sleep, we wake up — but that alone does not allow us to thrive, just survive. If we don't plug our phone in then it will never recharge. And I think that we must discover what it is that recharges us, what allows us to thrive and not just survive.

So after much discovery and research and time, I came to understand the power of meditation. And I realised that that was the missing piece in my life. That was what was going to allow me to recharge, so that I could be the best that I could be. I thought for such a long time that the only people who meditated were linen-wearing, bearded incense burners, but I realised that that is not the case. The highest paid CEOs and professional athletes that I've worked with across the globe have many things in common. But the one thing that really stood out for me was that they all meditated.

When I got back from Kansas City, I decided to go away on a meditation retreat, just for two days, to understand how meditation could serve my needs. And I must say that it has had a huge impact on me and my ability to continue to perform at my optimal level with the extensive travel schedule that I have — more than 180 flights in 2019 alone, across 22 different countries. And I think it's because I am now in much greater control of my mind that I can remain optimistic, resilient, courageous and healthy.

SOMETIMES
THE GREATEST
PAIN

✳ BRINGS US ✳
THE GREATEST
GLORY.

(14)

BECOMING A DAD

I've been very fortunate to achieve some wonderful things, learn some great things, and hit some milestones that people have told me I would never be able to. But I believe so powerfully that it's not about proving other people wrong but, more importantly, proving ourselves right. And there is a distinct difference between the two.

Without a doubt, the thing that I wanted to achieve, more than anything in the world, was to one day become a dad. That's the reason why we actually opened an orphanage. Because I wanted to understand what it felt like to be able to devote your love, your energy, your time and your emotion to children who look up to you, and admire and respect you. But also to keep you accountable for what you stand for, for what your visions and values are — and I know that without a doubt the greatest gift that God can bestow on any of us is to become a parent.

With all the ongoing health challenges that I've had throughout my life, this is the one thing the doctor said would never happen. However, through science and maybe a little miracle, I got the gift of becoming a father. Mel and I decided to go down the IVF path and we were hoping it would go like this: first round, baby arrives, happily ever after. However, we quickly realised that was not going to be the case. We underwent many, many rounds over many years, with incredible expenses associated, and we just couldn't make it happen. Not only was the emotional torture so tough for us, but what made it really tough was when we would go out in public and people would ask us, 'So guys, when are you going to have a baby?', not knowing that we were desperately, desperately trying to become parents.

I remember one day, two years into the process, when we thought that the IVF had worked: all the signs were looking good, and we really thought that we were going to be parents. But unfortunately at the nine-week mark we found out that we'd lost the baby. That afternoon we went to the coffee shop down the road and friends of ours walked past, gave us a hug, asked us how we were, and then again asked, 'So, come on you two, when are you going to have a child?' You can imagine my beautiful wife and I just broke into millions of pieces.

But finally, after many years of trying, the miracle occurred. We announced to the world in August of 2017 that we were expecting a baby. The media attention was overwhelming and we happened to get on many different TV shows, radio programs, magazines and newspaper articles, sharing the gift and miracle of being pregnant.

The lead-up to the arrival of our child was very smooth. Everything seemed to be going according to plan, and Mel was very healthy, very cautious of what she was eating. I was doing my best as a husband to minimise stress and get ready for that spectacular day when our child was to enter the world. We didn't know what sex the baby was because we wanted it to be a surprise.

Our little baby was due to arrive the end of February 2018. We decided to throw a huge baby shower at our house with all our friends and family to celebrate what was going to be the most remarkable gift that my family had ever received. My wife had set up photo booths, guessing games…you name it, she had organised it. The place looked beautiful, and the day was spectacular. It was so special to celebrate what was about to occur with our nearest and dearest.

About a week after the baby shower I was asked to host an event for a friend whose brother was running from Melbourne to Brisbane, raising money for a charity that I had never heard of before: the Miracle Babies Foundation. Once I started researching the charity before hosting the event I realised it was a really great organisation that aligned beautifully with what I stand for: helping to serve those that are in need. They develop and provide vital programs and resources to support and enhance a family's experience from a threatened pregnancy, to a hospital journey with a premature or sick newborn, to the transition to home and beyond. We raised a lot of money on the night and it was great to do something for someone else expecting nothing in return, but boy was I naive. How quickly that act of kindness would be returned, and in such an emotionally powerful way. We had no idea of the pain we were about to enter, and the fear that was about to take over our life.

I was travelling extensively all around the world and finally I had returned home the afternoon of 7 December. Mel was outside in the back garden with the hose pressed up against her back.

I asked, 'What's wrong?' And she said that she had experienced a lot of back pain that day, and the only thing that made it feel better was a pressure hose with cool water. I thought that didn't sound right (not that I know what's wrong and right —we were guessing as much as anybody). We had been going along to many different baby classes and prenatal classes and had met some really beautiful people who have now become lifelong friends. We contacted them and asked them if they had experienced anything like it, and they all said no.

So, we decided the next morning to head to the hospital to get some tests done. Everything seemed to be okay; the doctor assured us that everything looked fine and there was nothing to worry about. Before we were about to leave, she said she wanted to do one last internal review.

Which resulted in our world turning upside down. She informed us that Mel was 2 centimetres dilated and that we needed to jump on the emergency care plane from Coffs Harbour down to Sydney, as she was not yet 30 weeks pregnant.

I tried to stay as calm as I could, but internally I was absolutely freaking out. I was sent home to pack a bag full of clothes because they warned us that we could be in Sydney for upwards of 10 weeks until our baby arrived. In the rush of packing I didn't realise what I was actually doing—for myself I packed some comfortable clothes, some swim shorts, some normal day-to-day outfits. But for my wife, not thinking and freaking out, I packed all her work clothes. So Mel was going to be in hospital for up to 10 weeks and all I had packed was her suit jackets and work dresses, which no longer fit her! Which obviously wasn't going to work.

I arrived back at the hospital to find Mel strapped in the removal bed. We headed to the airport, and I remember just trying to keep her calm, explaining to her, 'Everything will be OK.' We arrived in Sydney at the Royal Hospital for Women in Randwick. Mel was examined and settled in. The following day she was having some lunch and the pain intensified, and they told us that it looked as though our baby was on its way. Mel was told to remain calm and flat on her back, and after some pain medication she seemed to settle in for the night with not too much discomfort. I slept on a thin mat on the floor next to her because I didn't want anything to happen without me being there.

It's crazy when you're in those situations, because I recall thinking to myself, 'This is the most uncomfortable bed I've ever slept on, and it's cold, and it's noisy.' Yet my wife was lying next to me in serious pain. Where was my perspective?!

The tenth of December was a very quiet day, with no major issues, lots and lots of rest, and card games. But the eleventh was action packed. Mel's waters broke and they thought our little baby was on its way. However, after the waters broke everything seemed to cease. And what was incredible was that Mel didn't even look pregnant after the waters broke. They said that this was very common based on the gestation of our baby and the size — again, nothing to really worry about.

And then the twelfth came rolling in. This was the day our world changed forever. Mel went into serious labour at around

6 pm. At the time I was actually out, going for a run. When I got the call, I immediately headed back for the hospital — I've never run so fast in my life. When I arrived, I walked straight in and said, 'I'm so sorry but I need to have a shower. I can't be down the business end smelling the way I am when our baby enters the world.' After 40 minutes of intense labour our beautiful little baby entered the world. Bang on 6.40 pm. They put our baby into a plastic bag because the skin was not yet formed completely. They asked me whether I knew what the sex was. I had not a clue, so I went to put my hand inside the bag and they said, 'No, no please don't touch the skin. Just look through the bag.' As I pushed between our baby's legs, to be really honest with you I thought it was a vagina. I said to Mel, 'We've had a girl!' But when I removed my hands from the groin area I saw a little doodle flop down. I was over the moon that I was the father of a beautiful little boy named Lachlan James Crossland.

The morning of our son's arrival, I had been asked whether I would like to go and look into the intensive care unit, which is where our baby would be heading once it was born. I told the doctor that I'd spent a majority of my life in hospital and didn't think that it was necessary. However, they insisted, so I decided to go and have a look. They took me through the three levels. On level 1, many of the babies were on the rebound and going very, very well. In fact, most of them were about to head home. Still, they were very small babies and it was quite confronting. Then they took me to level 2. Many of these babies had cords up their nose and needles in their hands. It was pretty intense. Finally they took me into level 3, where many of the babies were incredibly unwell. Surgeons were operating on children, their skin was not developed, and I remember the doctor saying to me, 'This is not where you want to bring your baby because many of these babies will never go home.' I immediately walked out of there because I was an absolute mess.

Once Lachlan was born, after putting a respirator on his face they escorted him into intensive care. I remember holding out my finger through the bag and his tiny hand gripped onto it. As we walked through the hallways heading to intensive care, at every bump we went over, my little boy squeezed my finger tighter. We arrived into intensive care and I hoped with every part of my heart that we were going to turn left and go into level 1. But we walked past that door, and past level 2, and straight into level 3. I can't tell you the fear and the pain that I felt. I literally collapsed to the floor. A big Irishman was there; he came over and put his arm around me and put me on his seat. He said, 'Mate, stay strong. And if you need a hug, I'm here for you.'

No sooner did I sit down and get my breath back than I saw a lady walking towards me. Her facial expression was almost soothing and calm. She put her hand on mine and said, 'Michael, my name is Barb and I am the CEO of the Miracle Babies Foundation. I am so grateful for what you have done for our charity and we will do everything we can to help you and your little boy. Stay positive and believe in your heart that everything will be okay.'

I couldn't believe how quickly a random act of kindness to host an event for a charity I had never heard of only weeks earlier had led to that very charity serving my needs, offering counselling, education and love to families with premature babies. I felt so blessed. It's amazing the impact that being reassured can have on us. Barb didn't know my son's complications. But it just gave me a sense of peace and inner belief that in fact everything would be OK.

They connected Lachlan up with every cord you could imagine, started pumping him full of drugs. They put him in a glass incubator — the only way we could touch our boy was through the holes in the side. Around 40 minutes later they wheeled Mel down; she had not yet seen our little boy, and she just fell to pieces to come into that room and see him with all those cords and needles. We were both incredibly broken because we had no idea of the severity of his illness.

Our little boy arrived at 30 weeks and he was not in good shape at all. Yet every single day the doctors were just overwhelmed with his progress. On day three, the doctors gave us the greatest news we had heard: we were finally allowed to hold our little boy. This tiny little baby. To see him in the arms of his mum was one of the most beautiful moments of my life. I captured a beautiful photo of our little boy holding onto his mummy as she looked down at him, a tear trickling down her cheek. And I don't think it was a tear of pain or sadness, but rather of joy. A tear that had been sitting in her heart for so many years of wanting to become a parent, and now finally she was holding her little boy.

After two weeks on level 3 they finally transitioned him to level 2, which was a huge step for his health and for our mental health. We were staying with friends and travelling to and from the hospital every single night because we weren't allowed to stay in the intensive care unit.

One day we went down to have a juice and sit in the sun while Lachlan was sleeping. We saw a lady whose little baby girl had been in the crib next to us in level 3; she was with her daughter, holding her in the sun, and I said to Mel, 'That's so unfair that she's allowed to have her little baby girl downstairs in the sun getting fresh air and we weren't allowed to take our boy even out into the hallway.' I couldn't help myself — I went up to the doctor that afternoon and said, 'Please, can we take our little boy outside? Just to let him see the sun and feel the warmth and breathe the fresh air.'

He said, 'Sorry Michael, no, he cannot.'

I couldn't help myself: 'That's so not fair. There's a lady who was next to us in intensive care level 3 who took her baby out this morning to get some fresh air. I just want to take him outside, just for a moment, to hold him in the sun.'

His reply shook me to the core. He said, 'Michael, we hope one day that you can take your little boy home. That woman will never take her girl home.'

Again, perspective is such a powerful, powerful thing. Sometimes we must just step out of our own shoes and look at life through somebody else's eyes to realise how blessed we are.

We tried to make the best of a tough situation. Every time our little boy was asleep we would go into the parents' room and talk to the other parents, have a great time, play cards and every other game you can imagine. We would listen to their stories and their pain and we would share ours. It was a really special place with wonderful people who actually have walked in your shoes. (Speaking of shoes, don't worry: Mel didn't spend the entire time in hospital walking around in business attire. After I'd made such a hash of packing for the hospital, we ended up couriering a bag of more suitable clothes down.)

After four weeks we got some great news: the doctors were going to fly our little boy back to Coffs Harbour. We didn't tell anybody because we wanted it to be a huge surprise. We boarded the air ambulance and flew back to Coffs Harbour with so much excitement in our hearts. Our little boy was going to spend the next four to six weeks in hospital in Coffs Harbour until he was fighting fit and ready to go home. We arrived at the hospital, gave our little boy a kiss and headed home for the first time in a month.

We invited our family and friends around to celebrate the life of our little boy and the fact that we were one step closer to bringing him home. That night after everybody left, my wife sat in the nursery, already all set up, and I noticed that the emotion on her face had changed from joy and happiness to fear and sorrow. She began to worry and wonder why we just couldn't have our little boy home. And she literally sat in the rocking chair for hours just staring at the empty cot.

Until we received a phone call from the doctor, saying, 'Michael you need to come in real quick.' I must say it was probably the fastest trip I've ever had from my house to the hospital. The doctor took me into one room and Mel went to our little boy's side to hold his hand. The doctor said to me, 'Michael, we are sorry to tell you this but we believe your boy has contracted an illness called sepsis, which is a blood disease. And with someone so fragile as your little boy the chances of him making it are very, very slim. His condition could deteriorate rapidly and he could be gone within the next four or five days.'

I have never felt that sort of pain before. I had aches and pains all over my body instantly. We were immediately airlifted back to Sydney and I experienced something that I hope no parent ever has to experience. I watched a doctor massage my son's chest as he had stopped breathing. I remember praying aloud on that plane, saying, 'God, take my house, take my car, take everything that I've ever earned in my life. But please, please don't take my little boy.'

We arrived back into Sydney and they sent us to Sydney Children's Hospital in Randwick. We were hoping and praying that we were going back to the Royal Hospital for Women in Randwick because they were incredible there. However, we arrived at Sydney Children's and we waited for 45 minutes in the waiting room with the ambulance officer as they tried to find us a bed. They were not aware of our arrival, which I think was insane. It was as though they had never dealt with a patient who was so little, and so young and so unwell.

We finally got put into a room and I remember the nurse saying to us, 'We can't really hear his machine going off from our station. So if he has any cardiac issues just give us a yell and we'll come straight in.' This meant that we could not leave his bedside — and we didn't, for nearly 42 hours, until I'd just had enough and I went over and begged and begged and begged the doctors at the Royal Hospital for Women to please take our little boy back. I said that I would do anything.

The next day the transfer papers arrived and we were allowed to take our little boy back to the Royal Hospital for Women, back to intensive care unit level 3. Instantly a sense of calmness washed over me. Four days after learning that he had sepsis, we captured his first little smile. And I truly believed in that moment that everything was going to be okay.

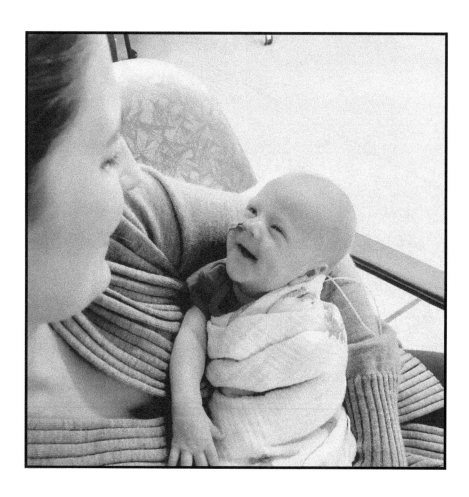

The day our son Lachlan James Crossland smiled for the very first time.

I needed to keep my mind active while in hospital, otherwise I was going to go insane. I identified after speaking with many doctors and nurses that medication was being stored three flights of stairs from where we were situated. I also noticed that a lot of the mums' expressed milk could not be stored as they did not have big enough fridges or freezers. It was absolutely remarkable what the mothers went through to express milk at all hours of the day and night to be able to provide for their babies, only for it to go to waste.

I was fortunate enough that I had a little bit of media attention and was asked to go on a very popular morning show in Australia called *Sunrise*. I thought that this might be a really wonderful opportunity to not only share our story but to also enlighten people and make them aware of the challenges that the hospital was facing and also the opportunity for them to help.

So I started a GoFundMe in hopes that we could raise enough money to buy some industrial fridges and freezers to be able to store not only life-saving medication but also all the expressed milk that these mothers were producing. The show aired on a Thursday morning. By Friday afternoon we had raised over $30 000 and were able to buy the industrial fridges and freezers.

People said that it was crazy, that in my darkest hour I still tried to find ways to help. I don't think that it was crazy on my behalf; I think it was a coping mechanism. I believe that we all deal with things differently, and the way I deal with adversity is to try and keep my mind active, keep busy and strive to serve other people to make an impact on their lives. And in this situation it did exactly that. It helped me keep my mind busy and it helped me truly make an impact on the lives of people I may never meet.

Through some of the dark days in hospital I began to realise I was finally getting a chance to feel what it was like, just for a moment, to walk in my mum's shoes. And I realised, so quickly, that it is far easier to be lying in the bed than standing next to it. It gave me such a sense of gratitude and appreciation for what my mum did for me. But also it gave me a greater understanding of the pain and suffering that she must have felt throughout all those years.

But she never ever gave up on me. And I was never ever going to give up on my little boy. We would sing to him, we would read to him, we would lay by his bedside and hold his finger until the doctors would ask us to leave for the night. The highlights of our days were when we were finally allowed to take him out of the humidicrib and have him lay on our chest. To feel his skin on ours and to hear his heartbeat was just indescribable. Once again, our little boy just got stronger and stronger, healthier and healthier. And he transitioned from level 3 down to level 2 and finally, after many weeks, made it to level 1. We knew that this was the place to be. And this got us one step closer to heading home.

Finally, the day came when the doctors said, 'Michael and Melissa, we are delighted with your son's progress. You can finally take him home.' I think we cried all the way back as we went to pack our bags and run back to the hospital. We were ready to go, and we were so excited to have our little boy back home. They airlifted us back to Coffs Harbour Hospital where he spent two nights before we were finally allowed to bring our little boy home.

The drive home from the hospital was the slowest drive I have ever driven in my entire life. I think I pulled over four or five times, just to make sure that he was OK.

We can now fast forward two years and he is a healthy, happy, gorgeous little baby. And I am so grateful every day that he looks like his mum and not his dad. What's incredible is he poos more than we could imagine. And he eats more than we could imagine. But I must tell you, we love our boy more than we could ever imagine.

Many say to me, 'Michael, you have been dealt with some really shit cards.' And I respond always with the same line: 'That just means I'm still in the game. And while I'm still in the game, how I choose to play those cards allows me to live a remarkable life.'

I've begun to realise over the many years of hardship and adversity that great darkness gives us our discovery moment. We do not discover how unfair our life is, but rather we discover how powerful we have been made.

SOMETIMES WE
PRAY TO CHANGE
THE SITUATION,

BUT WE
MUST
REMEMBER,
SOMETIMES
**THE
SITUATION
IS HERE TO
CHANGE US.**

(15)

DEALING WITH FEAR THROUGH FAITH

I am sure you would agree that in my life there have been many challenges to deal with, hurdles to jump and mountains to climb. But using the tools I have shared in this book has helped me to keep getting back up when the world has told me to stay down. I love the saying, 'They tried to bury me but they didn't realise I was a seed.' Not only have I realised what tools we must use to keep moving forward, but I also have identified that we must deal with fear through faith. And not so much a biblical faith, but something more like self-belief.

Fear can consume and cripple us, but I think when we learn to harness the fear and have it be our driver it can be huge. When we can shift our fear into our faith we can be dynamite.

Sometimes a situation occurs in our life that makes us think on a deeper level than ever before. I'm sure you've had this!

Once I was on an incredibly turbulent flight — so much so that the pilot spoke to all the passengers once we had landed, letting us know that it was the worst flight she had flown in over 20 years. Let's just say our stomachs were in our throats and many of the sick bags were full.

It got me thinking about the power of fear and the importance of faith. I had complete faith that the pilot would get us down safely, which helped to reduce my fear. I have faith that my driver will get me safely to my event, and so often in my life I have had faith that the doctors and surgeons would get the job done! It's amazing: we have no idea what type of day they've had, or how they are feeling emotionally and physically, yet we have faith in them, which helps us reduce our fear.

The one person we are in control of — the person who does control our emotions, our actions and who can get us through situations of fear — is the one person we often don't have faith in. That's the person who looks back at us in the mirror each day.

There is a saying about social media that 'we spend our life comparing our behind-the-scenes pain and suffering to other people's highlight reels'. And then we wonder why we have anxiety, fear and insecurities about the life we live.

We must have faith in who we are; we must have faith in our actions and behaviour; and we must have faith that the dots of life will eventually join up. Pushing through the barrier of fear will lead us to that ultimate destination.

Understanding what fear is, and not only analysing it but finding ways of dealing with it, can be a game changer. We all face and deal with different types of fear at various stages in our lives. Through research and self-discovery, I believe there are four stages of fear throughout our life:

- Early childhood: fear of strangers and fear of separation. This is unfortunately something my son struggles with as I am regularly away. When I'm home I can go to the toilet or into my office, and as soon as I am out of sight he loses it and starts to cry ...

- Childhood into adulthood: fear of specific objects (animals, insects — for me it's snakes) and also scenarios (such as thunderstorms, the dark).

- Adolescence: fear centres on social experiences such as humiliation and loneliness. I struggled with this a lot at school as I went from a primary school of 28 kids to a high school of 1200 and didn't really know anybody. I was a loner, and I found it hard to make friends and fit in; it took a long time before I found my people.

- Adulthood: we have much more abstract fears, such as the fear of failure.

But is fear really a bad thing? What is the message being communicated by fear? Is there a powerful learning behind the fear that we are feeling?

Fear is not necessarily a bad thing; it is one of the inbuilt human survival instincts. Too much fear, which paralyses action, is obviously the bad kind of fear. But have you ever done something you were fearful of doing then looked back and wondered why you were scared? I remember being too scared to jump off the jetty in Coffs Harbour. Finally, after what felt like 10 hours (which was probably more like 10 minutes) I took the leap of faith. When I landed in the ocean, my first thought wasn't 'I'm still so scared' — it was 'Let's do that again!' I wonder if there is something holding you back from being the best version of yourself. Maybe if you took that leap of faith then you'd reflect and think, 'Why didn't I do that years ago?'

Most people already know and are aware of the types of fear they face. Common fears are fear of:

- rejection
- change
- losing
- the unknown
- dying
- public speaking.

(On a side note, can you believe that on a list of 10 the number two most feared thing is dying, and the number one thing is public speaking? Which basically means most people would prefer to be lying in the coffin than reading the eulogy.)

Ironically, there is also fear of success, but I think the big one is the fear of failure... We get so scared of failing that we choose to not set any goals. I always remember that we learn far more from a loss then we will ever learn from a win. I certainly have a fear of failure, and as a result I push myself harder and set higher targets for myself so that the effort exerted and progress becomes worth it. Sometimes fear can point out the inadequacy that we have or what tools, skills, knowledge or abilities we lack to progress on a desired course of action. Fear acts as an alarm clock, reminding us that we need to do a bit more homework to pass the exam.

Being afraid makes you imagine all sorts of awful outcomes and scenarios. Sometimes the fear can be intense to the point of inaction, which is where people literally get stuck! But all we need to do is take that first step. Persevering through and in spite of fear stems from a determination to succeed and make a difference in your life and the lives around you.

Here are my top three reasons why fear is a really good thing when harnessed with faith:

1. Heightened awareness. At the basic level fear guides our fight or flight responses and helps to keep us safe and alive. Fear heightens your senses and awareness; it keeps you alert and helps you be prepared. To achieve great potential or greater heights, have fear and still push through it. Overcoming fear is done through action.

2. Acknowledgement and enlightenment. Taking time to understand what makes us fearful can yield useful insights and help us to prepare for the fear and even work on reducing the fear or the fear triggers. Learn from your past fears. Know that everyone faces fear at one

time or another; the fact that others have faced fear and persevered should motivate and encourage you.

3. Removal of barriers. Fear forces you to examine the real or imagined barriers that are holding you back. Removal of the barriers is not a one-off process — rather it involves identifying the major barriers holding you back and taking small steps and actions on a regular basis towards defeating the barrier. This really helps when you are dealing with the fear of the unknown. This gives us an opportunity to find someone who has been through it before; it allows us not to feel all alone and reinforces that we are not crazy.

I think that it's so important that we remember, 'The greater the obstacle, the greater the glory in overcoming it.

When I have fear around a goal, which I think is something we will all experience in our life, I ask myself three questions to help me process. Before asking the three questions I write on one side of a piece of paper the downsides of allowing fear to rule me around my dreams or goals. Then on the other side of the page I write down the upsides of moving through fear and taking back control. To see this written down helps get some clarity.

For example, say you're in a toxic relationship. Your downsides might be the fear that you are never truly going to be happy, fear of being alone and of hurting your partner. Your upsides might be being free, being able to breathe again and getting your life back.

Or say you're in the corporate world and you're thinking of leaving it. The downsides could be losing a guaranteed income and leaving your workmates. The upsides could be stopping the spiral of earning and spending, and being able to find yourself again.

Once you've gone through this exercise, go a little deeper and ask yourself these three questions:

1. What is the worst that can happen?

2. What are the benefits of doing it? Visualise the benefits of achieving it like it's already a done deal to give you excitement and insight into the feeling of succeeding.

3. Will you regret your decision not to act later?

Clarity around our feelings towards failure, success and regret actually frees our mind to think more clearly and act far more effectively. It gives us confidence and allows us to have a renewed faith in our direction, the goals and visions we have set and the belief that we can achieve anything. Having faith is a powerful tool; it can increase our confidence, drive and energy levels to help us go after our goal. When we start to believe in ourselves and what we have set out to achieve, our confidence will grow and our chance to succeed will skyrocket.

So it's great to process fear by going through the steps I've just outlined. In dealing with fear I also regularly use the move, share and help steps discussed in chapter 12.

I also like to sit in the space of fear. What I mean by that is a visualisation technique that has really assisted me in somewhat dissolving fear from my stomach. I think when we have fear and anxiety, rather than sitting in that space we try and push it away. In doing so, we don't push it away — we just push it deeper into our subconscious mind and it manifests into something far bigger than what it was when it initially entered.

The best example I can use here is when you have an argument or issue at work, and then all of a sudden you feel like everyone in the office is looking at you, everyone is talking about you, and you're under the microscope. But it's so not true. We think we are bigger and more important than what we really are and we need to get through it, over it, around it — however you want to go, but just get going.

I simply like to visualise the anxiety or fear as soon as it arrives, not suppress it. I focus on my breathing (breathing in for four, holding for two, breathing out for four and holding for two) and I like to work out what colour it is, how heavy it is, where it's sitting in my body. Then I speak with affirmation, telling myself 'Everything will be OK, it's far too light to weigh me down, I will get through this.' Give it a go next time you are feeling a little fear or anxiety; you'll be surprised how much it helps, and also how much quicker you get over things. I always remember that one of the greatest causes of cancer is stress, so let's minimise stress and anxiety at all costs.

The biggest difference I've noticed between successful people and unsuccessful people isn't intelligence or opportunity or resources: it's the faith and the self-belief that they can make it happen.

We all face difficulties, problems and setbacks in life. Some people have faith in themselves and they choose to move on against all the odds. Others believe that they can't do it or that their problems are bigger than themselves. What you choose to do is up to you. But one thing I know for sure is that your faith and self-belief say a lot about who you are and what your life will ultimately look like.

It's important we remember fear will do its best to distract us. But faith will look within us and will show us truly how powerful we have been created.

My mum had faith in me all those years ago. She pushed through the fear, the pain and the suffering to never give up on her dying son. Now here I am standing, fighting and doing my best to serve other people and leave a legacy. If you think you can't, then you are right; but if you think you can, you're also right. Don't dramatise your fear and allow it to take away your faith in yourself.

Remember, the sad news is that life is short...but the great news is you are the captain. Take control of your life, be accountable for your actions and take your world to new heights. We all have one life — this is not a dress rehearsal. Tomorrow is not guaranteed for any of us, so don't wait until it's too late before you take your first step in the right direction ...Now is the time!

I BELIEVE THE MAJOR CAUSE
OF UNHAPPINESS IS NEVER THE
SITUATION BUT YOUR
THOUGHTS ABOUT
THE SITUATION!

EMBRACE
THE CHALLENGE,
EMPOWER
THE MIND
& SMILE.

(16)

TOOLS TO SHIFT
YOUR MINDSET

Many people ask me how I manage to stay so positive and upbeat through some of the dark days. I use a very simple, yet effective tool: it's all about living above the line. Below the line is the Victim, and above it is the Navigator.

This principle can apply to your business, your personal life, your relationships, your challenges and your adversities. This principle is something you can use in every single part of your life. I promise you that all the people you look up to in the world, whether they are a public figure or not, live this principle that I am about to share.

If it is the only thing that you take away from this book, you will become a better human being if you can grasp this and apply it each day with your partner, children, friends, and even your staff. Everyone will notice the difference and will thank you for it.

OWNERSHIP
ACCOUNTABILY
RESPONSIBILITY

ARE YOU A
NAVIGATOR?

ARE YOU A
VICTIM?

BLAME
EXCUSES
DENIAL

IT'S NOT ABOUT HOW <u>OFTEN</u>
YOU SPEND ABOVE THE LINE,
BUT FOR HOW <u>LONG</u>.

I will start with below the line. I'm sure you can relate to this stage. When we are below the line, we generally lie in BED:

- **Blame:** We don't mean to do it or want to do it, but we simply do. We always want to point the finger, forgetting that when we point the finger, there are always three of our own fingers pointing back at us. Typically, when things are not going smoothly, when happiness is low, relationships are tough and frustration is high, we tend to stay in this space.

- **Excuses:** We all do this every single day of our lives. We procrastinate, we come up with reasons why we didn't succeed, why we didn't have a go, and why we didn't try just one more time.

- **Denial:** Denial is the trickiest one to truly understand or identify, because we don't know when we're in denial. It takes someone who respects us and cares about us to say, 'Hey, this is what I see happening in your life.' If you drink a lot of alcohol, the fact of the matter is you are probably an alcoholic, but for you, it's just a few six packs each night after work. It's going to take someone who cares about you to say, 'Hey, it's time to slow it down a bit', and for you to listen to what they are telling you. Otherwise, something is going to happen to your liver, you're going to be in trouble, and it might be too late. So don't get to that place.

Any time you Blame someone, make Excuses or are in Denial about a situation, you are what we call a Victim.

Nevertheless, life is full of choices: you have the choice to spend your time below the line, or you can stand up. You can break the barriers down and truly embrace living.

The word above the line is OAR:

- **O**wnership: Own that whatever happens is about you, your choices, your actions, your behaviours, etc.

- **A**ccountability: Have some accountability for each decision, action and outcome that is delivered.

- **R**esponsibility: We have an obligation that if we truly want to become the best version of ourselves, we must take responsibility for our life.

With your OAR you can steer your ship in the direction you want to take and get the results in life you want. You can have the love you want from your family, you can have the relationship you want with your children. If you want certain things in your life, which we all do, you need to spend the bulk of your time above the line.

Still, sometimes you feel as though you're on a paddle boat with one oar, and you're paddling so hard to get ahead in life, but really, you're just going around and around in circles. So rather than working smarter and getting some support, or even using a tool such as this one, you work harder until eventually you're completely and utterly exhausted. When you have no more time and energy to give, you spiral out of control and you live your life as a Victim.

The people who live above the line are called Navigators. These are the people you see on TV, in sport, in the arts, and in business. I think we all want to live above the line and we want to earn the right each day to live in this space. This is where we all need to be.

It's important to understand that we all go below the line — every one of us, every day — but it's not about how often you go below the line. It's about how long you stay there. When I was 26, I nearly gave up. Due to health challenges that were mounting again, I just stayed in BED mode. It took all of my power away and all of my confidence. Still, I made choices in my life and took ownership and responsibility for my wife, my mum, my family and for myself. I wanted a brighter future, I wanted to bring inspiration and hope to the world, and I wanted to help make changes in individuals each and every day.

How would you address your challenges in both your professional and personal world differently if you were above the line? How would you use the resources you have at your fingertips more effectively? How would you interact with your family, friends and clients? How would you view the objections and excuses from the people around you?

For all of us to keep bouncing over obstacles, we need strength and determination, but we also need tools, because we all have bad days, moments and situations in our life that can drag us below the line into the Victim space. In those times I have my mother, my family and my inner belief that I am on this earth for a great purpose.

It's amazing how some people make life seem effortless and simple. They achieve amazing goals with seemingly no struggle, breeze through the hardest days without breaking a sweat, and they seem to be happy, even in the toughest of circumstances. These people are not different from you. In fact, they face the same feelings and anxieties. However, what separates the successful and the unsuccessful isn't genetic material or ability, but their mindset. They choose to stay above the line, they choose to be positive, and they choose to grab their OAR and steer their life in the direction they choose!

We all know that life is in our hands and we control the outcomes of every adversity, every challenge and even every victory. A wise man once said, 'Do not allow success to go to your head nor failure to affect your heart.' We will always learn far more from a loss than we will ever gain from a win. We can choose to see obstacles in front of us as a mountain too steep and not worth climbing, or we can see it as another great challenge. Brick walls are not there to keep us out; they are there to show us how bad we really want it!

Let's look into the mindset of a Victim and a Navigator in more depth.

No doubt, everyone knows someone who thinks their life is just too hard; they constantly complain and freely share with you how unfair their life is. It's always someone else's fault why they are failing, unhappy and even depressed. It may be a friend, a work colleague, a family member, or it may even be you. It's important that we are honest with ourselves, that we can put our hand on our heart and be truthful to who we are, where we are and what we wish to become.

Some people feed off being a Victim and love the sympathy that is given when they are in a dark place; they don't want to change and they don't feel that they deserve to live a better life. When you're in this space, you are stuck in BED: you just want to pull the covers up over your head and to shut out the entire world.

Some phrases you might say as a Victim:

- I can't do that.

- Life is just not fair.

- I wish life would just give me a break!

- Why me?

- My life is so unfair!

- I'm stuck counting my problems.

This creates a mindset shift, and your entire world feels darker, duller and destructive. So, your mind sees things like:

- the glass always being half empty

- a difficulty in every opportunity

- just not enough hours in a day

- it can't get much worse.

Some real-life and simple examples of a Victim's mentality that we all experience each day include:

- That would be right, trust me to get the red light!

- Far out, you've got to be kidding, its only 11 am. Why is this day dragging out?

- I'm in the eight items or less aisle and that painful person in front has at least 10 items. Who does she think she is?

- It's not my fault I'm late to work. How was I supposed to know that traffic would be bad?

- You just cut me off; did you not see my two-tonne, four-wheeled, bright red car heading into your lane?!

When we are below the line, we forget that life is supposed to be enjoyable, and that every day is truly a gift that needs to be embraced and treasured. But, as we all know, life is all about choices and those choices can reshape, re-mould and redefine our future.

Let me give you an example of when I recently became a Victim. I just finished a large speech in Melbourne at a national nurses conference with over 400 in attendance. A speaker's rating is 0–5, with a score of 5 being outstanding and rarely achieved across the professional speaker world. I received a 4.87 and my agent called and informed me it was the highest score he had seen. With over 300 completed surveys and comments, this was something I should be very proud of. So I decided to read all the comments, and was really enjoying them — but out of the 300, the one negative comment just sucked me in and consumed my thoughts. The comment read, 'Too Americanised, and far too evangelistic for my liking.' I couldn't help myself: all I could focus on was the one bad comment as opposed to the 299 good ones.

To stop playing the Victim card, and begin to live in the Navigator space, we need to grab our OAR — take Ownership, Accountability and Responsibility — so we can take our life to new heights. You know when you are in this state of mind as you want to spring out of bed: you're excited about each day and are really engaged with life.

Some phrases you will say when being a Navigator:

- Could be worse...

- I'm facing a few challenges, but nothing I can't handle.

- I'm loving life and all that it throws at me.

- I'm so lucky every day.

- I enjoy counting my blessings.

These phrases, in turn, shift the mindset, and now your entire world feels brighter, clearer and happier. Your mind sees things like:

- the glass always being half full

- an opportunity in every difficulty

- laughing to shift your mood and your mindset to cope with challenges

- the ways your life is great

- awareness of when you dip below the line and become a Victim, and bouncing back.

Some real life and simple examples of a Navigator's mentality that we all experience each day include:

- Its only 11 am, so there's much more time to get things done.

- Wow, I hope that the person who cut me off is OK; clearly, they're in a rush.

- It's not the adversity I'm facing, but rather how I deal with it, so I'll be fine.

- Who can I help today to make their life better?

As mentioned earlier, a very important and powerful point with this principle is: 'It's not about how often you become a Victim that determines the health of your mindset, but rather, how long you stay there.' You can become a Victim 50, 70, 100 times a day.

However, as long as you identify yourself as dipping below the line and spring back above the line, the quality of your life, your mind and your future will improve out of sight.

This principle will, no doubt, assist greatly if you maintain accountability and work to be in control of your mind. However, the 10 habits that follow have enriched and empowered some of the biggest stars on the planet; their simplicity might surprise you, and they are not just habits, but tools that you can embrace along your journey.

I believe these 10 points can be the key to your transformation, along with mastering your mindset and living above the line.

1. **Set yourself unique and inspiring goals every single day.**
    Jerry Seinfeld is one of the world's most celebrated comedians. He's also one of the richest. Since the final episode of *Seinfeld* aired in 1998, he's earned $3.1 billion in repeat fees. Seinfeld's success didn't come out of thin

air. Instead, he used a remarkably simple productivity system to come up with the best jokes and funniest stories: every day, he would write something. It could be a single joke, a funny anecdote, or even a full episode's script. After he'd finished writing, he would mark the day on a wall calendar with a red X. After a few days, a chain of crosses started to emerge on the calendar. Seinfeld's only goal was to keep the chain going every day. Whether it was a Monday or a Sunday, he sat down to write, and marked each day with a big red X.

2. **Before you sleep, summarise your biggest achievements.**

   There's more to productivity and success than just setting goals. After all, it's easy to set goals and then ignore them. Before you go to sleep, look back over your daily to-do list and cross off tasks you've completed. Add any incomplete tasks to the next day's schedule and force yourself to complete them.

3. **Wake up at the exact same time every day.**

   Everyone knows the importance of going to sleep at the same time every night. Few people, however, know how important it is to wake up at the same time every day. Set yourself a 'wake-up time' and make sure you're alert, awake, and out of bed at the right time each morning. Whether you go to sleep at 10 pm or 4 am, make sure you stick to your schedule. Waking up at the same time every day helps to set your circadian rhythm — an internal body clock that keeps your body energetic, healthy and focused.

4. **Don't fall for multitasking.**

    You've probably heard how important multitasking is
    for getting things done. Here's a little secret: it's really
    not that great. Multitasking sounds like an excellent
    strategy for getting work done — after all, what could
    be better than doing two tasks in the time it normally
    takes to do one? Its only problem is that it doesn't work
    far more often than it does work. The world's most
    successful people all have one thing in common: they
    focus on one goal at a time. The world's best CEOs
    and artists always achieve one goal before starting
    on the next.

5. **Don't spend too much time online.**

    Most people waste a huge percentage of their work
    day online. Even if you're focused and attentive at
    work, you doubtlessly spend at least an hour or
    two browsing Twitter and Facebook once you get
    home. It's amazing what you can achieve when you
    dedicate time normally spent on social media to
    achieving your goals and transforming your life. Log
    off early and go for a run, develop your artwork,
    spend special time with your family or expand your
    dream business!

6. **Practise mindful eating for health and relaxation.**
    Mindful eating is a Buddhist practice that asks you
    to do something simple: eat your food slowly and

appreciate every single bite. It sounds silly, but it's an amazing way to do two things: eat a better diet and truly appreciate the taste of the food that you eat. Next time you're about to stuff down dinner, stop and appreciate the taste, the smell and the texture of your meal.

7. **Every week, reconnect with a friend or acquaintance.**

   In France and Italy, workers take two-hour lunch breaks to socialise and reconnect with their friends and co-workers. In Hong Kong, businesses refuse to answer their phones from 12 pm until 2 pm due to the importance of taking time off for lunch. Does your rushed, fast-paced lifestyle make it difficult to sit down with friends and acquaintances for lunch? Set yourself a goal of catching up with friends every week for an extended lunch or dinner; your mind and body will appreciate it.

8. **Write down your thoughts before you go to bed for a great night's sleep.**

   Do you spend hours tossing and turning before you fall asleep? There are hundreds of reasons for insomnia to occur, but one of the most common is anxiety over your thoughts. Purge your mind of demanding thoughts by keeping a special diary on your bedside table. Whenever you find yourself worrying about something, write it down to deal with tomorrow. Not only will this help you fall asleep faster, you'll also wake up feeling refreshed, prepared, and ready to conquer last night's thoughts and ideas.

9. **Eliminate negative people from your life.**

   Some people are emotional vampires. These people feed on your happiness and seem to drag you below the line whenever you're feeling happy with your life. Lifelong Victims can be emotional vampires and a huge drag on your happiness, your focus and your ambition. Write them out of your life to feel more focused and ambitious, as well as far more in control and happy.

10. **Avoid technology an hour before you go to sleep.**

    Technology is addictive, and using it too much (or for too long) can lead to tech burnout. Free yourself from tech addiction by turning off your computer, tablet, phone and TV at least an hour before you go to sleep. Not only will this give you some personal time to reflect on your day or read a new book, it will also help you to fall asleep quicker. Some researchers believe that using screens before sleeping stops your body from producing melatonin, which is an important sleep hormone.

I think that it's important to attempt just three habits that resonate with you right now as the ones that you need to implement and master first; we should never try to master all 10 at once. Otherwise, you will become overwhelmed and not change anything. I try to remember something that I learned from Dr John Demartini:

When you invest in you, the world will invest in you. When you begin to love you, then the world will begin to love you, and finally, when you value you for the person you are and the difference you can make, the entire world will begin to value you.

THE
LONGER
WE DWELL
ON OUR PAST
MISFORTUNES,

THE GREATER IT
DAMPENS THE
EXCITEMENT
FOR OUR
FUTURE.

⑰
WHERE TO
FROM HERE

My health is a continual challenge. People ask me all the time how my health is and my response is always the same: Mentally, I'm in a great space. I think that as long as we are mentally strong then the days we are fortunate enough to spend on this earth will be days that we can truly enjoy because our minds are in the right place.

Recently, I had a melanoma scare, where they had to do a lot of work on my face. (Sadly it didn't make me look better, ha ha.) Fortunately they removed all the issues and right now I am delighted to be cancer free.

I'm sure you would agree that sometimes we try to deal with things by ignoring them. But, whether the problem is personal or professional, this is not the way to go about it. A small issue swept under the rug can eventually turn into a massive trip hazard. We must embrace the challenges that we face head-on and strive to be in the mental space that we need in order to overcome life's challenges.

I'm incredibly grateful for the life that I live. I dearly love my wife. I'm incredibly grateful to be a dad and have a beautiful healthy little boy. I'm so blessed to be surrounded by wonderful people who continue to see me stretch and grow to become the best me that I possibly can be.

In 2019 I flew on 180 flights across 22 countries around the world. I'm an ambassador for many different organisations, including Camp Quality, the Cancer Council, the Lyme Disease Association of Australia, Hope for Haiti, and the Make-A-Wish Foundation, and I've been the Australia Day ambassador for the best part of a decade. However, despite being able to achieve little milestones here and there, I continue to get told what I can't do in life — and I love showing them that I can.

* * *

At the time of writing, it is the start of April 2020. The world is filled with fear, anxiety and uncertainty as we face a pandemic like never before. Tens of thousands of people around the world are dying from COVID-19, with the figure rising every day. Unfortunately, my tenuous health places me in the high-risk category for this virus, so I am thankful for the controls and constraints imposed by our government. I am also deeply grateful for the care and common sense of the many thousands of strangers who are vigilantly following the health and safe distance protocols in order to stem the spread of the pandemic and protect the vulnerable in our community.

This worldwide pandemic has seen the closure of many thousands of businesses. Millions have lost their jobs, and life today has no resemblance to life even a month ago. Gyms, parks and beaches are closed, and we are unable to hug friends or shake hands. We must stay at least 1.5 metres away from each other, and if we are seen in public with more than two in a group, we are fined on the spot and risk being arrested. The world as we know it has changed forever, and it is in these uncertain times that we must focus on the emotional and psychological health of every individual, stay positive, stay in the present, and take the time to connect with our family. There is so much work ahead of us, but the worldwide community is resilient.

I have no doubt that our world will rebuild and recover, however it is my wish that this recovery will bring with it the opportunity for us to re-evaluate and reset our priorities. I hope that we enter a new era where we more fully appreciate the little things that so many of us took for granted for so long: a hug, a meal at a restaurant, social interaction with friends, a picnic in the park and time with family.

For many of us who have never lived through wars or depressions, we are experiencing an unprecedented level of human devastation, and one that will require an unprecedented level of resilience from us all.

I have watched the closure of friends' businesses, I've seen the heartache of having to postpone weddings and other family celebrations, and I've stood by in support as friends have lost their jobs. Professionally my entire year of events has been cancelled: my roadshow with Tony Robbins is cancelled, as is my USA tour as tour manager with the Australian Expos team.

When Mel said to me, 'What are we going to do?', my response was simply, 'Everything will be OK.'

* * *

There are a number of ways you can connect with me on social media and the web, which include:

Website: www.michaelcrossland.com

Facebook: facebook.com/MichaelCrosslandcom-112483922154060

Twitter: twitter.com/mikecrossland

LinkedIn: au.linkedin.com/in/michaelcrossland

Instagram: www.instagram.com/michaelcrossland

Videos: michaelcrossland.com/videos

CPSIA information can be obtained
at www.ICGtesting.com
Printed in the USA
JSHW041056231122
33721JS00003B/4